The Unbreakable

Mind

The Unbreakable

Mind

Proven Strategies to Strengthen Your
Cognitive Power with Lifelong Clarity

Dr. David Brainard

Contents

Introduction 1

Chapter 1: Understanding Neuroplasticity 5

Chapter 2: Strategies for Cognitive Enhancement 13

Chapter 3: Nutrition for a Healthy Brain 21

Chapter 4: The Impact of Exercise on Brain Health 28

Chapter 5: The Role of Sleep in Cognitive Performance 35

Chapter 6: Stress Management and Mental Resilience 41

Chapter 7: Mastering Focus and Concentration 49

Chapter 8: Memory Enhancement Techniques 56

Chapter 9: The Power of Lifelong Learning 63

Chapter 10: Mind-Brain Relationship: Insights and Applications 71

Chapter 11: Creativity and Brain Function 79

Chapter 12: The Aging Brain: Myths and Facts 87

Chapter 13: Social Interaction and Brain Health 94

Chapter 14: Technological Interactions and Brain Health 101

Chapter 15: The Role of Positivity in Cognitive Health 108

Chapter 16: Understanding Brain Injuries and Recovery 115

Chapter 17: Brain Health Myths and Misconceptions 123

Chapter 18: Future Directions in Brain Research 131

Chapter 19: Tailoring Cognitive Strategies for Individuals 139

Chapter 20: Enhancing Emotional Intelligence 146

Chapter 21: The Role of Genetics in Brain Health 153

Chapter 22: Cognitive Impacts of Drug Use and Recovery 160

Chapter 23: Influence of Environment on Cognitive Health 168

Chapter 24: Brain Health and Lifestyle Design 175

Chapter 25: Evaluating Brain Training Programs 182

Conclusion 189

Introduction

In an age defined by rapid technological advancement and ever-increasing demands, the pursuit of brain health, cognitive enhancement, and personal development has never been more pertinent. We find ourselves in environments saturated with stimuli, often overwhelmed by the very pace that promises progress. Yet, amidst this whirlwind, lies an incredible opportunity to harness the power of our brain—the epicenter of our thoughts, emotions, and actions. This book invites you on an enlightening journey to explore and unlock the latent potential resting within your mind.

At its core, this book is about empowerment. It's about understanding that no matter where you start, your brain's capacity for growth and adaptation is a remarkable constant. We often underestimate how our everyday choices, from what we eat to how we manage stress, can significantly impact our cognitive abilities. By incrementally tweaking these choices, you can craft a life that not only meets but exceeds your aspirations.

Imagine possessing the tools to enhance your memory, maintain mental agility, and ensure emotional well-being throughout the varied phases of life. This is the promise that understanding brain health holds. It's not a vague concept relegated to scientific circles but a practical arsenal anyone can use. Our intention here is to demystify the science and provide actionable strategies that fit seamlessly into everyday life.

The emphasis on neuroplasticity, the brain's ability to reorganize itself by forming new neural connections, forms the backbone of our exploration. This incredible characteristic of the brain ensures that you're never too old to learn, modify behaviors, or develop new habits. By delving into this subject, we accentuate hope—a notion that personal transformation is always within reach.

Cognitive enhancement isn't solely about boosting intellectual prowess; it's about leading a balanced life. Whether it's engaging in mindfulness practices to meditate and center yourself, understanding the impact of nutrition, or incorporating exercise into your routine, the goal is harmony between body and mind. This balance not only nourishes mental health but also drives sustained productivity and contentment.

Moreover, this book aims to dispel myths that often cloud our understanding of the brain. It provides clarity through evidence-based insights, allowing you to replace misconceptions with facts. The knowledge gleaned from these pages will enable you to navigate a world often filled with conflicting advice about brain health with confidence.

A significant aspect of brain health that we'll uncover is the idea of lifelong learning. The pursuit of knowledge need not end with formal education. On the contrary, adopting the perspective of perpetual learning enriches cognitive vitality, fostering a mindset that's open to continual growth. Learning is an enduring adventure, a boundless terrain waiting to be explored.

While technology and the digital age offer unprecedented access to information and connectivity, they also contribute to cognitive overload. In our exploration, we'll tackle the nuances of digital interaction and its impact on the brain. The aim is to strike a balance that leverages the positives of technology while mitigating its adverse effects.

The road to enhanced cognitive health encompasses understanding the integration of genetics, lifestyle, and environment. We'll discuss how these elements influence your mental capabilities and offer strategies to design a brain-friendly environment, minimizing potential risks. It's about creating conditions wherein your brain not only functions optimally but thrives.

Emotions and their interplay with cognition constitute another pivotal theme. Emotional intelligence can be honed just like any other skill, offering a substantial boost to your overall mental faculties. By understanding and managing your emotions, you can improve interpersonal relationships and lead a more fulfilled life.

This introductory glimpse only scratches the surface. As you delve deeper into the chapters, you'll encounter a comprehensive suite of tools and insights designed to enhance every aspect of your cognitive health.

Whether you're aiming to sharpen focus, enhance creativity, or maintain cognitive function with age, this book is here to guide and inspire.

The future of brain research is promising, with many breakthroughs on the horizon. This book will also shed light on these advancements, giving you a peek into the future of cognitive science. Emerging technologies are poised to revolutionize our approach to brain health, and staying informed can only serve as an advantage.

We invite you to embark on this journey with an open mind and an eagerness to discover the untapped resources within yourself. Remember, enhancing brain health isn't just about acquiring knowledge; it's about applying it in ways that transform how you live, interact, and grow. Let's create a world where we not only survive the mental challenges but excel in every capacity of our lives.

Chapter 1

Understanding Neuroplasticity

In the fascinating landscape of the human brain, neuroplasticity stands out as a beacon of hope and potential. It's our brain's extraordinary ability to adjust, reorganize, and form new connections, even as we age. Picture this: we have within us the capability to reshape our minds based on experiences and learning. It's like an internal workout, where our neurons are the weights, and with each 'rep'—whether it's acquiring a new skill or adapting to a change—we strengthen our cognitive muscles.

Understanding neuroplasticity not only explains why we can bounce back from setbacks but also highlights the endless possibilities for personal growth and cognitive enhancement. By harnessing this potential, we can improve our brain health, enhance our capacities, and truly transform our lives. It's less about being stuck with what we've been given and more about unleashing the power we all hold within.

The Science of Neuroplasticity

Neuroplasticity, a term that might sound more at home in a lab than a living room, is a captivating, transformative force within our brains.

At its core, neuroplasticity is the brain's astonishing ability to reorganize itself. This incredible capacity for change allows our central nervous system to adapt to new experiences, environments, and learning processes, essentially enabling the brain to rewire itself. It's the scientific underpinning of how we learn new skills, recover from brain injury, and form both short-term and long-term memories. In recent years, scientists have begun to appreciate just how powerful and pervasive this capability truly is, pointing toward numerous applications in cognitive enhancement and personal development.

Let's peel back the layers of neuroplasticity a bit further. To understand the cellular ballet that allows for such dynamic change, we must look at neurons, the brain's building blocks. Neurons are interconnected through synapses, which are like tiny bridges over which information traverses. Each time we learn something new or have a novel experience, these synaptic connections either strengthen or form anew. This is synaptic plasticity, a critical component of neuroplasticity, playing a big role in memory and learning. Through repeated activation, some neural pathways become more efficient while others weaken due to lack of activity. This synaptic reshaping equips us with the ability to adapt our skills and memories as life's demands evolve.

The idea of a "hard-wired" brain is now antiquated, thanks to groundbreaking research illuminating the ways neuroplasticity operates across our lifespan. Previously, it was thought that significant brain change was confined to childhood, after which the brain was set in a fixed pattern. Modern neuroscience has shattered this myth, revealing that adults, too, possess a high degree of plasticity. This means rapid learning, adaptation to new environments, and recovery from injury are possible long after the brain's formative years. This ongoing capability provides hope and potential avenues for interventions in conditions like stroke and degenerative diseases.

Despite its robust nature, neuroplasticity isn't always a friend. In some instances, it can foster negative patterns. For example, when exposed to stress or trauma, the brain can adapt by strengthening pathways related to fear or anxiety. Similarly, maladaptive habits may become ingrained, as the brain efficiently wires itself to prioritize familiar, albeit harmful, behaviors. Recognizing these potential pitfalls of neuroplasticity is just as important as understanding its positive aspects because it helps us find ways to influence it beneficially.

This quirky brain rewriting feature doesn't operate in isolation. It's part of an intricate dance involving chemical signals known as neurotransmitters. Dopamine, for instance, plays a vital role in motivation and reward- driven learning. When you're learning something intriguing or achieving a goal, dopamine floods the synapses, reinforcing the patterns that led to these outcomes and encouraging the brain to repeat them. This dopamine- related boost can make learning addictive in the best possible sense.

Likewise, acetylcholine helps direct attention, enhancing the ability to learn and remember new information. These chemicals are the brain's internal cheerleaders, guiding the process of neuroplastic change.

A particularly exciting area of study within neuroplasticity involves its implications for recovery. Consider stroke rehabilitation. When a stroke damages part of the brain, regions that were once responsible for functions like speech or movement can be compromised. Through targeted therapy and exercises, other parts of the brain can be retrained to take over these roles, a process made possible by the brain's innate plasticity. This adaptability underscores the importance of creating supportive and stimulating environments for individuals seeking recovery, as these can catalyze the brain's healing processes.

Another fascinating element of neuroplasticity is its enhancement through various lifestyle choices and practices. Cognitive exercises and new learning experiences, of course, encourage neuroplasticity, but so do meditation and mindfulness practices. Research indicates they can boost cortical areas involved in attention and emotional regulation, thanks to the brain's reorganization ability. Physical exercise also enhances neuroplasticity, promoting neurogenesis — the creation of new neurons — particularly in areas associated with memory and learning. What we eat plays a role, too, as certain nutrients and superfoods can fuel and support structural changes in the brain, enhancing plasticity.

So, why is understanding neuroplasticity so essential? The awareness of its mechanisms and potential opens doors to cognitive enhancement that can transform personal and professional lives. By intentionally engaging in activities that promote positive neural rewiring, individuals can sculpt their brains, thus expanding capabilities in focus, memory, and reasoning. It becomes a proactive endeavor, shaping the architecture of our minds to better handle the complexities of modern life, all while fostering resilience against cognitive decline.

In summary, neuroplasticity is more than a scientific curiosity; it's a fundamental principle of change, adaptation, and growth within our brains. As we delve deeper into understanding this incredible capability, the potential for improved brain health and cognitive function becomes not just an aspiration but an accessible reality. Through adaptive learning, deliberate practice, and lifestyle choices, we hold the remarkable power to influence the ways our minds function, proving that, indeed, it's never too late to teach an old dog new tricks.

Benefits of Neuroplasticity

Neuroplasticity, the brain's remarkable ability to reorganize itself by forming new neural connections, stands at the forefront of brain health and cognitive enhancement. Understanding its benefits can be transformational. Before diving into specifics, it's important to grasp the sheer potential that lies within our brains. This dynamic process not only shapes who we are but also empowers us with an unparalleled capacity for growth and change.

One of the immediate benefits of neuroplasticity is cognitive flexibility. Imagine your brain like a complex city with highways and backroads.

When one route becomes unavailable, another opens, allowing traffic to flow to its destination. Similarly, neuroplasticity helps your brain reroute information, adapt to new situations, and learn novel tasks. This capability can significantly enhance problem-solving abilities and creativity, turning challenges into opportunities for innovation.

For those facing recovery from injury or illness, neuroplasticity is a beacon of hope. When areas of the brain are damaged, whether from trauma, stroke, or degenerative diseases, other parts of the brain can learn to take over lost functions. This compensatory mechanism enables recovery by forging new pathways and reinforcing different areas to support cognitive functions, providing a pathway to regain lost abilities and independence.

Memory is another domain where neuroplasticity provides profound benefits. By regularly engaging in activities that promote brain plasticity, such as learning a new language or playing a musical instrument, individuals can improve their memory retention and recall skills. This enhancement isn't just temporary. Continued engagement ensures long-lasting improvements, maintaining a sharp and agile mind for years to come.

The advantages of neuroplasticity also extend to emotional health. The brain's ability to change doesn't only apply to cognitive processes; it affects emotional regulation as well. Through practices like mindfulness and meditation, individuals can actively rewire their brains to foster a greater sense of well-being, reduce stress, and enhance emotional resilience. This transformation leads to healthier relationships and an improved overall quality of life.

On a broader scale, neuroplasticity supports lifelong learning. It is the foundation of education, giving our brains the capacity to absorb new information and skills at any age. Contrary to previous beliefs that cognitive decline is an inevitable part of aging, neuroplasticity proves that the brain remains capable of growth throughout life. This capacity empowers individuals to pursue new interests, embark on different career paths, or simply continue to learn for personal enrichment, making lifelong learning a reality rather than just a concept.

For those struggling with maladaptive behaviors or ingrained habits, neuroplasticity offers a pathway to change. By understanding how habits form and implementing strategies to create new, healthier pathways, individuals can overcome addictions, negative thought patterns, or unproductive habits. This ability to reshape behavioral patterns highlights the empowering and transformative nature of neuroplasticity, enabling personal development and growth.

One often underestimated benefit of neuroplasticity is its role in enhancing attention and focus. In today's fast-paced world, the ability to concentrate on tasks without being distracted is more valuable than ever. Neuroplasticity aids in strengthening the neural networks associated with attention, allowing for improved focus, better task completion, and increased productivity. This improvement not only boosts professional performance but also enriches personal pursuits.

The social aspect of neuroplasticity is equally remarkable. Engaging in social activities and building meaningful connections can stimulate brain plasticity, enhancing cognitive functioning and emotional health. These interactions encourage the development of new pathways and support the maintenance of a vibrant and active mind, reducing the risks associated with isolation and cognitive decline.

Furthermore, neuroplasticity plays a vital role in adapting to new technologies and environments. As the world evolves with technological advancements, our ability to learn, adapt, and proficiently navigate digital landscapes becomes increasingly important. Neuroplasticity empowers us to harness technology for cognitive enhancement while also ensuring that we can adapt to environmental changes, safeguarding our brain health in an ever-changing world.

In conclusion, the benefits of neuroplasticity are vast and far-reaching, touching every aspect of our lives. From cognitive flexibility and recovery from injury, to memory improvement, emotional health, lifelong learning, and social interaction—neuroplasticity is the powerhouse enabling change and growth. Understanding and embracing these benefits not only enriches our lives but also equips us with the tools necessary to thrive in a dynamic and unpredictable world. So, let's harness the power of neuroplasticity for our cognitive enhancement and personal development, turning the potential within our brains into reality.

Chapter 2

Strategies for Cognitive Enhancement

Building a sharper mind doesn't require a revolutionary breakthrough; it can begin with small, deliberate actions that fit seamlessly into your daily life. In this chapter, we dive into practical strategies that empower you to enhance cognitive function through simple yet effective methods.

Engaging in cognitive exercises accelerates mental growth, pushing your brain to build new pathways and strengthen existing ones. Mindfulness and meditation techniques train your brain to focus and reduce stress, improving both clarity and creativity. Whether incorporating puzzles, learning a new skill, or simply breathing mindfully, these strategies can transform everyday moments into opportunities for cognitive rejuvenation. Welcome to a journey where unlocking your brain's potential is as accessible as it is rewarding!

Cognitive Exercises for Mental Growth

Engaging in cognitive exercises is like setting off on an exciting quest for mental growth. These exercises go beyond merely playing games; they're about actively nurturing and stretching the brain's capabilities. Whether it's adult life or childhood, cognitive exercises form a central part of our journey toward improved brain function and mental agility. Like a workout for the brain, they demand effort but surely deliver rewards in clarity, speed, and creativity. Through repeated engagement, they also encourage neuroplasticity, helping the brain adapt and develop throughout an individual's life.

The beauty of these exercises lies in their ability to fit any lifestyle. From apps designed to test memory and problem-solving to board games that challenge strategic thinking, the possibilities are endless. Each activity can target specific areas, like working memory or lateral thinking, ensuring a well-rounded mental flex. However, consistency is key. Just as you wouldn't expect to build muscle after a single workout, don't expect mental growth overnight. Making cognitive exercises a habitual part of your daily routine can lead to gradual but noticeable improvements in cognitive performance.

Consider puzzles, for instance. Jigsaw puzzles enhance spatial reasoning, while crosswords boost linguistic capabilities. By solving puzzles, you tap into logical reasoning and pattern recognition, crucial skills that can be applied to real-world scenarios. The beauty of puzzles is that there's a fit for everyone, from those who prefer quiet solo tasks to those who enjoy family game nights. Plus, these activities stimulate different parts of the brain, making them a comprehensive tool for cognitive enhancement.

Cognitive exercises don't always need to be formal or structured. Everyday activities, like learning a musical instrument or practicing a new language, also double as excellent mental workouts. When you learn a new skill, you're challenging your brain to forge new pathways and connections. This not only improves memory and cognition but can also Lead to an increased IQ. The process of learning can be frustrating, but the benefits make every stumble valuable.

Reading is another powerhouse activity for mental growth. It traverses different forms, from novels to non-fiction. Each type challenges the brain in unique ways, fostering empathy, understanding complex concepts, and enhancing vocabulary. The practice of reading demands focused attention and often involves complex thought processes like synthesizing information, predicting plots, and analyzing characters.

Moreover, reading regularly can slow cognitive decline, making it a lifelong gift you can give your brain.

Technology can also be harnessed effectively. Brain-training apps provide users with a plethora of activities specifically designed to boost cognitive abilities. From Lumosity to Elevate, these apps cater to a variety of cognitive domains, such as attention, flexibility, and problem-solving. They provide immediate feedback, allowing users to track progress and adjust exercises to better suit their evolving needs.

Socialization, though often overlooked, acts as a cognitive exercise, too. Engaging in conversations, playing team sports, or participating in group activities requires quick thinking, attention to detail, and robust communication skills. Social interactions force the brain to process information rapidly while also requiring emotional and cognitive empathy. This assists in maintaining a healthy and responsive brain, thus proving the saying that humans are social creatures at heart. Regular social engagement can delay mental decline and provide a refreshing mental stimulus that solitary activities sometimes can't offer.

Mindfulness and meditation, while extensively discussed in the next section, deserve brief mention here. They serve as cognitive exercises by honing attentional focus and emotional regulation. Practicing mindfulness aids in improving working memory and can result in more profound cognitive flexibility. When combined with other mental exercises, mindfulness can magnify the benefits, ensuring a balanced approach to mental fitness.

Finally, one mustn't forget the importance of play. Play isn't just for children; adults benefit greatly too. Engaging in creative, spontaneous play stimulates the brain in remarkable ways, fostering innovation, problem-solving, and resilience. Activities could include theater, creative writing prompts, or simply experimenting with different artistic media without worrying about the final outcome. Allowing space for error and novelty within the realm of play challenges the brain to adapt and grow continuously.

Mixing various cognitive exercises keeps the brain engaged and continuously learning. By maintaining this variety, you prevent boredom and ensure that multiple cognitive domains are being simultaneously improved. Explore different activities, switching between solitary tasks like reading or apps and social ones like board games with friends. Keep it fun—after all, the journey to mental growth should be as enjoyable as it is beneficial.

In conclusion, cognitive exercises are integral to nurturing a sharper, more agile mind. From the subtle joys of reading to the structured challenges of brain-training apps, these activities offer numerous pathways toward enhanced cognitive function. Remember, the brain is a muscle that thrives on exercise and growth. Embrace a mindset of lifelong learning and consistent practice, and you'll find your mental landscape becoming richer and more resilient with time.

Mindfulness and Meditation Techniques

Like the gentle ripples that spread across a pond, the practice of mindfulness and meditation can bring about profound changes in cognitive enhancement strategies. When you focus on the present, allowing yourself to be fully immersed in the moment, you open up pathways in the brain that can boost your mental faculties. These practices offer a gateway to mental clarity, reduced anxiety, and improved concentration. The hustle and bustle of daily life can cloud our thoughts, making it difficult to harness the full potential of our minds. Mindfulness creates a refuge from this chaos, a place where we can cultivate our cognitive abilities with care and attention.

At its core, mindfulness is about paying attention. But it's not just any attention. It's a deliberate focus on the present moment, accepting it without judgment. By doing so, we slowly train our brains to become more efficient and aware. This practice is essential for cognitive enhancement because it helps us break free from the constant barrage of distractions that compete for our attention. A study published in *Psychological Science* showed that regular practice of mindfulness can lead to improvements in working memory, focus, and even academic performance.

Let's take a closer look at meditation — often seen as the sibling of mindfulness. While mindfulness can be practiced in the moment, meditation requires setting aside time to achieve a deeper state of relaxation and awareness. There are many forms of meditation, each catering to different cognitive needs. Transcendental Meditation, for instance, involves silently repeating a mantra to settle the mind into a state of profound rest. In contrast, mindfulness meditation focuses more on breathing and observation, leading to increased awareness as well as emotional regulation.

Mindfulness-Based Cognitive Therapy (MBCT) serves as a prime example of how these techniques can be integrated into cognitive enhancement. Originally developed to prevent relapse in depression,

MBCT incorporates mindfulness to help individuals break negative thought patterns. It demonstrates how blending traditional techniques with modern psychology can foster enhanced cognitive function, promoting greater mental strength and resilience.

Practicing mindfulness and meditation doesn't require a complete lifestyle overhaul. Start small. Perhaps carve out a few minutes in the morning, before checking your phone or diving into your daily tasks. Use this time to sit quietly and focus on your breathing. With consistency, this practice can become as ingrained in your routine as brushing your teeth. Feel the rhythm of your breath, notice the subtle sounds around you, and gradually, you'll find your mind sharpens, your emotions stabilize, and your overall well-being improves.

Another powerful technique is progressive relaxation. This method involves tensing and relaxing different muscle groups in the body, fostering a sense of deep relaxation. When practiced regularly, it can enhance our focus and awareness, making it a potent tool for cognitive enhancement. By alleviating physical tension, our mental clarity can flourish, akin to cleansing a fogged mirror to reflect more clearly.

But how does one measure the tangible effects of these practices? Research over the years has consistently supported the cognitive benefits of these practices. Neuroimaging studies show that meditation can lead to structural changes in the brain, particularly in areas linked to attention, emotion regulation, and self-referential processes. The thickness of the cerebral cortex can increase with regular practice, improving focus and decision-making capabilities.

Another noteworthy aspect of these techniques is their accessibility. No fancy equipment is required. You don't need to visit an exclusive retreat or purchase expensive gear. All it requires is your dedication and a willingness to embrace the present with an open heart. Your cozy cushion at home or even a quiet corner in your office can transform into a powerful space for meditation. These practices can accompany us in our everyday tasks, helping us approach challenges with a refreshed mind and a balanced perspective.

Mindfulness and meditation can also become communal practices. Engaging with a group can provide support, shared experiences, and motivation to persist when the initial excitement wanes. Moreover, group meditation sessions can enhance the collective energy, making individual practice even more rewarding. Learning from others' experiences can also offer fresh insights into how these practices can further augment cognitive functions.

As you embark on or continue this journey, remember that mindfulness and meditation are lifelong practices. They're not about achieving a permanent state of calm or unwavering focus but about cultivating the ability to return to the present moment when distractions arise. It's this returning, this practice of coming back to the breath, the moment, that holds the real power in enhancing cognitive functions.

Ultimately, by integrating mindfulness and meditation techniques into our cognitive enhancement strategies, we're nurturing not just our minds but our whole selves. These tools are like the strings of a finely tuned instrument, keeping us in harmony amidst the complexities of life. With each session, each breath, we stride towards not just a higher cognitive function but towards a more fulfilled and resilient state of being. So, embrace the journey, savor each moment, and watch as your mind unveils its vast potential.

Chapter 3

Nutrition for a Healthy Brain

As we dive into the world of brain health, it's essential to understand how nutrition plays a pivotal role in optimizing our cognitive functions.

Fueling our brains with the right foods is like giving a car the premium gas it needs to run efficiently. Foods rich in antioxidants, good fats, vitamins, and minerals provide energy and aid in protecting against brain diseases. This isn't just about eating right to improve focus and memory; it's about nourishing every part of our brain for long-term health and functionality. Imagine unlocking the brain's potential by simply making informed choices at mealtime—it's empowering! By incorporating brain-boosting foods into your diet, you can enhance mood, sharpen memory, and maintain a more agile brain as you age. Remember, a well-fed brain is a happy brain, and the path to cognitive excellence starts on your plate.

Essential Nutrients for Cognitive Function

Our brains, these incredible, complex organs that control everything we do, require a steady intake of nutrients to function optimally. Just like a car needs fuel, our brains rely on certain key nutrients to maintain cognitive function and overall brain health. Without these vital elements, we're like a vehicle sputtering along without premium gasoline. Let's delve into the specific nutrients that play a crucial role in supporting and enhancing cognitive capabilities.

Omega-C Fatty Acids: The Brain's Best Friend

Omega-3 fatty acids, particularly EPA and DHA, are perhaps the most renowned nutrients when it comes to brain health. These essential fats are critical components of brain cell membranes and are involved in cell-to- cell communication. Studies have shown that they can improve memory, enhance mood, and protect against cognitive decline. A deficiency in omega-3s can lead to impaired brain performance and development, making them essential for all ages. Fatty fish, such as salmon, mackerel, and sardines, along with walnuts and flaxseeds, are rich in these brain- supportive fats. If fish isn't your thing, fish oil supplements can be a useful alternative.

B Vitamins: The Brain's Energy Boosters

B vitamins, including B6, B9 (folate), and B12, play various roles in cognitive function. They contribute to the production of neurotransmitters, help control inflammation, and are instrumental in maintaining energy levels. Homocysteine, a common amino acid in your blood, can impair brain function when elevated, and B vitamins are key regulators in keeping these levels in check. Leafy greens, eggs, and legumes are abundant in B vitamins, making them vital additions to your diet for maintaining a sharp mind.

Antioxidants: The Protectors

If you picture oxidative stress as rust on a car, you'll appreciate the importance of antioxidants in keeping your brain free from wear and tear. Vitamins E and C, along with flavonoids, are powerful antioxidants that mitigate oxidative stress and inflammation in the brain. Blueberries, nuts, and seeds are excellent sources of antioxidants and have been shown to improve brain function over time. By incorporating these foods into your daily meals, you're not just fueling your body—you're shielding your brain from the damaging effects of time and toxins.

Choline: The Memory Aid

Choline often flies under the radar, but it's a powerhouse when it comes to memory and learning. As a building block of acetylcholine, a neurotransmitter crucial for memory and cognitive processing, choline is essential for brain function. Eggs are a superb source of choline, with the yolk providing the majority of this nutrient. Incorporating choline-rich foods like eggs or lecithin-based supplements can help bolster your brain's sharpness and memory retention.

Magnesium: The Relaxant

Magnesium's multifaceted role isn't just limited to muscle relaxation; it's also vital for brain health. It supports neuroplasticity, which is the brain's ability to form connections and adapt, crucial for learning and memory. Additionally, magnesium helps regulate neurotransmitters and supports a balanced mood. Foods like dark leafy greens, nuts, seeds, and whole grains can provide ample magnesium, ensuring that your brain is calm, collected, and ready to tackle new challenges.

Zinc: The Mood Stabilizer

Though more recognized for its immune-boosting properties, zinc also enhances communication between neurons and can influence the brain's response to stress and mood disorders. It's involved in the modulation of synaptic activity and neurotransmission. You can find zinc in foods like shellfish, meat, and legumes. Including zinc in your diet is a smart move for not just a sharper, but a more balanced mind.

Iron: The Oxygen Supplier

Iron is indispensable for ensuring that your brain receives the oxygen it needs to function. It plays a key role in producing red blood cells, which transport oxygen throughout the body, including your brain. With iron deficiency, you might experience brain fog, reduced productivity, and even impairments in learning. Foods like red meat, spinach, and lentils can boost your iron levels, ensuring that your brain remains well-oxygenated and alert.

Vitamin D: The Mood Enhancer

Technically a hormone, Vitamin D has been shown to impact brain health significantly. Low levels are associated with mood disorders, cognitive decline, and even some neurological conditions. Sun exposure is one of the best ways to increase Vitamin D, but fatty fish, fortified foods, and supplements can also help maintain adequate levels, particularly in the darker months when sunlight is scarce.

Adopting a balanced, nutrient-rich diet isn't just beneficial—it's essential for sustaining mental agility and resilience. The synergy of these nutrients acts as a foundation for brain health, supporting everything from mood stabilization to memory enhancement and more. As you embark on your journey toward better cognitive health, remember that what you choose to feed your brain today will affect its functionality and vitality in the years to come.

Brain-Boosting Superfoods

We've explored the essentials of cognitive nutrition; now, let's dive into the vibrant world of brain-boosting superfoods. These aren't just your average fruits and veggies; they're like the VIPs of nutrition, offering an array of benefits to keep your brain firing on all cylinders. Think of them as the secret weapons in your arsenal for enhancing mental acuity, focus, and even emotional health.

Contrary to what some might believe, brain food isn't confined to exotic ingredients or complicated recipes. Many of these powerhouse foods are staples you might already have in your kitchen. Take blueberries, for example. These little berries are packed with antioxidants, known to protect the brain from oxidative stress and may even reduce the effects of age-related conditions such as Alzheimer's disease or dementia. Throw a handful into your morning smoothie or oatmeal and you're already on the right track.

Then there's spinach, a leafy green that's been lauded for its potential to enhance memory. Rich in lutein, folate, and beta carotene, spinach is said to help preserve brain functions that decline with age. Pair it with some nuts and seeds - another superfood category rich in vital omega-3s and other essential fats - in a salad or as a snack, and you've got a brain- loving combo to envy.

Speaking of omega-3s, fatty fish like salmon, mackerel, and trout deserve a special mention. Their rich composition of eicosapentaenoic acid (EPA) and docosahexaenoic acid (DHA) is celebrated for promoting brain health and reducing neurodegenerative processes. Fish oil supplements can be an alternative for those not inclined to seafood. This is why they've earned the descriptor "brain food."

Don't overlook the power of green tea, which is celebrated in many cultures. Beyond its role in relaxation, green tea is rich in polyphenols and antioxidants, which are associated with improved memory and focus. The presence of caffeine and the amino acid L-theanine provides a gentler, more stable energy boost, helping to enhance brain function without the jitters often linked with coffee.

If you're the sort who's partial to nuts, you're in luck. Particularly, walnuts are a top-notch choice. Not only are they shaped like little brains, but they also boast high levels of DHA, a form of Omega-3 that can improve cognitive performance and help ward off stress. A few walnuts a day can make a difference; they're nature's way of offering a tasty snack with brain benefits.

Turmeric isn't just for curries - it's a brain superfood in its own right. Curcumin, the active compound in turmeric, holds promise in boosting BDNF (Brain-Derived Neurotrophic Factor) levels, which can delay or even reverse brain degeneration. Its anti-inflammatory properties potentially make turmeric a calming agent for the brain, providing benefits for memory and mood. Consider adding it to dishes, smoothies, or teas for a gentle cognitive nudge.

Dark chocolate is another indulgence that comes with brain perks. Containing flavonoids, caffeine, and antioxidants, dark chocolate is thought to enhance memory and boost mood. Plus, it's an anti-inflammatory, which helps with long-term brain health. Choosing chocolate with a high cocoa content reaps the best benefits, making it a sweet treat with significant advantages.

Don't underestimate the common bean, either. Filled with protein, fiber, and essential B vitamins, beans help with neurogenesis – the growth of new neurons. This makes them a fantastic plant-based protein source to ensure you're mentally sharp throughout the day.

Fermented foods might sound like an unusual addition to the list, but they're essential given their capacity to improve gut health, which is closely linked to cognitive function. Foods like yogurt, kimchi, and sauerkraut contain probiotics that help maintain a healthy microenvironment in the gut, which is essential for mental well-being.

Lastly, hydration plays a pivotal role in maintaining brain health. Consuming enough water supports mental clarity and concentration. But did you know that eating water-rich foods like cucumbers and watermelon can also contribute? They're refreshing and help keep your brain ticking without the hazards of dehydration.

The beauty of these superfoods lies in their diversity and accessibility. By incorporating even a few of these into your daily meals, you're actively crafting an environment where your brain can thrive. Whether through smoothies, salads, teas, or snacks, these foods offer flexible options to support cognitive health. A balanced approach ensures your mind stays sharp, your spirits stay high, and your future self remains grateful for the care you're investing today.

Chapter 4

The Impact of Exercise on Brain Health

Exercise isn't just about building muscles or improving cardiovascular health; it plays a crucial role in nurturing a healthy brain. Engaging in regular physical activity unleashes a cascade of biological effects that bolster cognitive function and overall brain wellness. When you exercise, your heart isn't the only organ that benefits—your brain does too!

Exercise increases blood flow to the brain, which in turn enhances the delivery of oxygen and nutrients. This boost helps improve memory, sharpens focus, and even promotes neurogenesis, the creation of new neurons. It's like a natural fertilizer for your brain. So, whether you thrive in high-intensity aerobics or prefer the steady rhythm of strength training, each drop of sweat is an investment in your brain's future, protecting against cognitive decline and elevating mental clarity. Make movement a cornerstone of your daily routine and watch as it weaves its magic, transforming not just your body, but your mind as well.

Aerobic Workouts and Cognitive Improvement

When you think about exercise, it's often about the physical benefits: losing weight, toning muscles, or building endurance. But what if there was a way to transform our perception and see it as a powerhouse for brain health too? That's where aerobic workouts come into play. These exercises, characterized by their rhythmic, sustained nature that demands increased oxygen consumption, aren't just heart-healthy—they're a cognitive goldmine. There's compelling evidence that aerobic exercises such as running, cycling, and swimming have an undeniable impact on our cognitive faculties.

Let's dive into the science behind this. Aerobic exercise affects the brain through increased blood flow, which means more oxygen and nutrients reach your bustling neurons. This strengthens the connection between different parts of the brain, essentially boosting creativity, enhancing problem-solving skills, and improving memory. The hippocampus, an area in the brain pivotal for learning and memory, is one of the major beneficiaries, growing as a result of aerobic activity.

Beyond just structural enhancements, aerobic workouts encourage the release of brain-derived neurotrophic factor (BDNF). BDNF acts almost like a miracle-grow for the brain, promoting the growth of new neurons and helping to maintain existing ones. It's a key player in the brain's plasticity or ability to adapt and form new connections, thus helping ward off cognitive decline as we age.

It's important to note that aerobic exercises don't require marathon-level commitment to be effective. Moderate, consistent involvement is key.

Activities like brisk walking, dancing, or even a lively game of basketball can be sufficient to gain cognitive benefits. The goal is to increase your heart rate and keep it elevated for an extended period.

Psychologically, the benefits are also significant. Regular aerobic activity helps to boost mood, reduce anxiety, and combat depression. How does this tie into cognition? When your mental health is stable, your cognitive functions tend to improve too. Better mood and reduced stress levels contribute to clearer thinking and better focus, making it easier to absorb and retain information.

What's incredibly motivating is that these benefits aren't confined solely to adults. Studies show that children and young adults who engage regularly in aerobic exercise exhibit enhanced cognitive performance as well. In schools, a short burst of physical activity can mean better focus and improved academic achievement.

Moreover, for those in the golden years of life, aerobic workouts might be particularly potent. As the natural decline in brain volume sets in with age, incorporating regular aerobic activities can help mitigate this process, maintaining cognitive functions well into the later stages of life.

In practical terms, defining a routine for aerobic workouts can make a world of difference. Start with simple steps—literally—by incorporating more walking into your daily habits. Park further from the store entrance, take the stairs instead of the elevator, or consider a daily stroll during your lunch break. Gradually build from there; your brain will thank you.

Consistency is the magic word here. While the initial motivation might be strong, staying committed is where many stumble. Find activities that excite you; maybe it's a dance class with friends, cycling through a favorite park, or even exploring virtual workouts online.

Remember, the goal is to foster a lifestyle change, one where aerobic workouts seamlessly integrate into your everyday routine. This doesn't mean you need to sign up for a gym membership or invest in costly equipment. The beauty of aerobic exercise lies in its simplicity—you can start now, right where you are.

Let's embrace this holistic view of exercise—not just sculpting our bodies but empowering our minds. The next time you lace up your sneakers or hop on a bike, envision each movement not just as a step toward physical fitness, but as a stride towards cognitive clarity and resilience.

In our bustling lives, where multitasking is the norm, giving our brains this form of exercise might be one of the best gifts we can offer ourselves. Let's take advantage of this simple, yet powerful tool to elevate not just our physical state, but boost our cognitive vitality and mental

well-being.

So go on, get moving, and unlock the potential within. The benefits of aerobic workouts for cognitive enhancement are within reach, and with each heartbeat, you're crafting a healthier, sharper, and more resilient brain.

Strength Training for Neuroprotection

When we think about exercise, especially strength training, it's common to picture toned muscles or increased physical fitness. But what if we told you it had profound implications for your brain as well? Yes, strength training doesn't just help build a brawny body; it plays a significant role in neuroprotection and overall brain health.

Now, let's dive into what makes strength training a valuable ally in maintaining and enhancing brain function. Strength training, or resistance training, involves exercises that improve strength and endurance by working against a force. This can be lifting weights, using resistance bands, or even performing body-weight exercises. These activities do more than just fortify muscles; they trigger a series of biological processes in your body that benefit the brain in unexpected ways.

One of the critical benefits of strength training is its impact on neuroplasticity, the brain's ability to adapt and rewire itself. When you engage in resistance exercises, the activity stimulates the release of growth factors. These are proteins that play a crucial role in the health of neurons, the cells responsible for transmitting information in the brain and body. They promote the growth and survival of neurons, encouraging the formation of new synaptic connections, which is essential for learning and memory.

More than just making the mind sharper, strength training appears protective. It contributes to neuroprotection—the preservation of brain health and function. As we age, the risk of neurodegenerative diseases, such as Alzheimer's and Parkinson's, increases. Interestingly, research suggests that consistent strength training might lower these risks or delay their onset. By bolstering synaptic connections and neuronal health, it creates a more resilient brain environment.

An often-overlooked benefit of strength training is its positive effect on mental health conditions like anxiety and depression. Engaging regularly in strength workouts helps regulate mood by boosting the production of endorphins, the body's natural painkiller and mood elevator. These hormones can alleviate feelings of anxiety and depression. But beyond the immediate emotional lift, there's evidence that strength training also fortifies the brain against stressors that can contribute to these conditions.

Strength training uniquely influences cognitive function. Unlike aerobic exercise, which primarily boosts cardiovascular health, resistance exercises increase levels of a protein known as brain-derived neurotrophic factor (BDNF). BDNF supports brain cell growth, survival, and overall brain plasticity. Higher levels of BDNF are associated with better cognitive function and mental agility, making strength training a formidable tool in enhancing mental performance.

The beauty of strength training is its accessibility and adaptability. No matter your age or fitness level, resistance training can be tailored to fit individual capabilities and goals. This inclusivity means that anyone can harness its neuroprotective benefits, paving the way for improved cognitive health and function. Whether you're lifting weights, engaging in Pilates, or using resistance bands, you're contributing to a healthier brain.

Don't forget the social aspects, either. Many strength-training programs occur in group settings, from gyms to community classes. These environments promote a sense of community and support, providing additional mental health benefits. The social interaction inherent in group workouts can help combat loneliness, which is itself a risk factor for cognitive decline. The encouragement of peers and shared goals bond individuals, creating a support system that enhances mental resilience.

What's crucial is incorporating strength training into your routine sustainably. Most experts recommend at least two to three days of resistance training each week, focusing on various muscle groups to ensure a balanced approach. By doing so, not only are you fostering a robust physique, but you're also investing in long-term brain health. It's the consistency that ultimately matters, and over time, the cognitive benefits become evident.

In conclusion, the benefits of strength training extend beyond the physical, reaching deep into the realm of cognitive health. By integrating resistance exercises into your lifestyle, you're adopting a holistic approach to wellness—strong muscles, a resilient mind, and a fortified brain. The insight here is simple yet profound: by strengthening the body, we also shield the brain against the challenges of aging, stress, and potential cognitive decline.

Next time you pick up a dumbbell or stretch that resistance band, remember that each movement is not just sculpting your muscles but is also a crucial step towards safeguarding your mental faculties. The mind-body connection becomes increasingly apparent through strength training—a true path to total health.

Chapter 5

The Role of Sleep in Cognitive Performance

In the hustle of modern life, sleep often gets shortchanged, yet it holds a cardinal role in sharpening our cognitive prowess. Picture this: during those precious hours of slumber, our brain engages in a flurry of activity, consolidating memories, clearing out toxins, and rejuvenating vital neural connections. Ignore sleep, and you risk impairing your focus, decision- making, and creativity, leaving your mental toolkit painfully dull. By embracing a regular sleep schedule and creating a calming bedtime routine, we can tap into the restorative magic of sleep. Not only does this improve our cognitive performance, but it also sets the stage for a more vibrant and healthy brain. So, let's not undermine the humble power of a good night's rest — because a sharper, more resilient mind awaits on the other side.

Understanding Sleep Cycles and Brain Rest

Sleep is one of those magical times when our bodies and minds repair, reenergize, and rejuvenate. But it's not just about getting a certain number of hours each night. To truly understand sleep's role in cognitive performance, we need to delve a bit deeper into sleep cycles and brain rest.

Let's start with the basics. Sleep is more than just turning off the lights and laying your head on the pillow. It consists of several stages that cycle throughout the night. These stages are broadly categorized into REM (Rapid Eye Movement) and non-REM sleep, and they have distinct roles in keeping your brain in top shape.

During non-REM sleep, which has stages 1 through 3, our bodies go from light sleep to deep, restorative sleep. In these stages, physical repair happens, and energy is replenished. When you wake up feeling refreshed, it's thanks to this essential deep sleep. Stage 3, often referred to as slow-wave sleep, is particularly crucial for brain rest as it helps consolidate memories and clear out irrelevant information. It's like your brain's physical decluttering and detox-time.

Then, there's REM sleep, the stage most associated with dreaming. It's fascinating because it plays a pivotal role in emotional regulation, problem-solving, and creativity. This stage of sleep provides a playground for your brain to process emotions and experiences that you encountered during the day. It's like a mental rehearsal, solidifying learning and enhancing cognitive performance. Without adequate REM sleep, you might find your memory a bit foggy, or your mood not quite where you want it to be.

Understanding these cycles is crucial because they don't happen in isolation. An entire sleep cycle, ranging from 90 to 120 minutes, repeats multiple times overnight. The more cycles you complete, the better your brain performs the next day. Skimping on sleep might mean missing out on crucial cognitive benefits that occur in these later cycles.

Interestingly, recent studies highlight how sleep cycles can vary dramatically between individuals, influenced by age, lifestyle, and even genetics. For example, teenagers naturally have a delayed sleep phase, meaning their biological clocks drive them to sleep later and wake later. On the other hand, adults tend to settle into a more consistent pattern, needing around 7-9 hours for optimal function.

You might wonder what happens if these cycles are disrupted. Well, research has shown that sleep deprivation negatively impacts cognitive abilities like attention, decision-making, and problem-solving. Even partial sleep deprivation—losing just some stages of sleep—can lead to significant deficits in alertness and cognitive performance. Chronic disruptions can even affect brain structure over time, leading to longer-term cognitive impairments.

The concept of "sleep debt" is particularly relevant here. Missing out on essential sleep stages can accumulate over time, similar to financial debt, and your brain will eventually demand repayment in the form of increased sleep need or drowsiness, particularly in restorative stages like slow-wave and REM sleep.

What's becoming increasingly clear is the link between quality sleep and neuroplasticity—the brain's ability to adapt and reorganize itself. High-quality sleep promotes the growth and strength of synaptic connections, driving learning and memory consolidation. Without sufficient sleep, these connections weaken, dampening cognitive functions and creativity.

The implications of understanding sleep cycles go beyond personal health —it can also impact workplace performance, educational outcomes, and general well-being. Organizations that recognize the importance of sleep schedules and brain rest could yield happier, healthier, and more productive individuals.

So, how can we leverage this knowledge for better brain health and cognitive performance? Prioritizing sleep hygiene practices such as maintaining a regular sleep schedule, creating a restful environment, and minimizing caffeine intake near bedtime can help optimize these sleep cycles. Such efforts ensure you hit the right balance between deep sleep and REM stages.

Nap strategically. Naps under 20 minutes can boost alertness without causing sleep inertia, while longer naps can help repay some of that elusive sleep debt, though timing them earlier in the day is best to avoid night-time disruptions.

In conclusion, the understanding of sleep cycles and brain rest isn't a mere bedtime story—it's a science crucial to unlocking our cognitive potential. We've only begun to scratch the surface on the intricate connection between quality sleep and enhanced brain performance. Let this chapter serve as a gentle nudge toward cultivating sleep as a non-negotiable pillar for cognitive health. Embrace the power of restful sleep, and wake up to a world of mental possibilities. It's not just about turning the switch off for the night—it's about preparing your brain for the wonders it can achieve tomorrow.

Tips for Improving Sleep Quality

Quality sleep is an indispensable cornerstone for bolstering cognitive performance. A good night's sleep doesn't just boost mood and energy; it sharpens attention, heightens creativity, and bolsters memory. Yet, with our hectic lifestyles and constant digital interactions, attaining that restful slumber can seem elusive. Fear not, as there are concrete steps you can take to elevate the quality of your sleep and thereby enhance your brain's capability.

First and foremost, consider establishing a consistent sleep schedule. Our bodies thrive on routine. Going to bed and waking up at the same time each day, even on weekends, can significantly improve sleep quality. This consistency reinforces our body's sleep-wake cycle, or circadian rhythm. *Disrupting this rhythm with erratic sleep patterns can make it difficult for you to fall or stay asleep.* Simply put, find a schedule that suits you and stick to it.

A calming pre-sleep routine can also work wonders. This might involve winding down with a book, practicing deep-breathing exercises, or enjoying a warm bath. Such activities signal to your brain that it's time to relax and prepare for sleep. **Avoid screen time at least an hour before bed**; the blue light emitted by phones and computers tricks your brain into staying alert by mimicking daylight, inhibiting the production of melatonin, the sleep hormone. So, try swapping your tablet for a paperback or indulge in some light stretching.

Your sleep environment plays a crucial role too. Ensure that your bedroom is conducive to sleep. An ideal sleep space is dark, quiet, and cool. Consider blackout curtains or sleep masks to block out light.

Earplugs or white noise machines can drown out disruptive sounds. *Keep your bedroom temperature comfortably cool*, around 60-67°F (15-19°C), which is often deemed optimal for sleep.

Another critical aspect is your diet. While a nighttime snack might seem tempting, steer clear of large meals and caffeine close to bedtime. Such indulgences can lead to discomfort and disrupt sleep. Instead, choose sleep-promoting foods like almonds, kiwis, or chamomile tea. These can soothe you into slumber without the risk of unwanted wakefulness.

Regular physical activity is a potent ally of restorative sleep. Engaging in vigorous exercise during the day can deepen sleep and help you sleep faster. The movement not only tires your body in a good way, but also reduces anxiety and depression, which are common culprits of restless nights. Just remember, timing is crucial; try not to exercise too close to bedtime, as this might keep you wired.

Yet, at the heart of these actionable steps lies the importance of managing stress. Stress and anxiety are among the most common sleep disruptors. Techniques like mindfulness meditation can help quiet an overactive mind. Practicing mindful breathing exercises or focusing on each part of your body melting into the mattress can lull you into sleep gently.

Cultivating a mindset of letting go and focusing on the present moment lightens your mind and readies it for rest.

Lastly, keep an eye on your napping habits. While naps can be refreshing, especially if your nighttime sleep was insufficient, long or irregular napping can confuse and disrupt your circadian rhythm. If you must nap, try to keep it short—around 20-30 minutes—and do it earlier in the day to prevent interference with your nighttime sleep.

By embracing these strategies, you're not just ensuring better rest but also an agile, more active mind. Good sleep habits support your efforts toward peak cognitive performance and mental clarity. Comprehensive cognitive enhancement relies on a holistic approach, and prioritizing sleep is a vital part of that journey. You deserve to wake up rejuvenated, ready to tackle the day's tasks with vigor, creativity, and focus.

Chapter 6

Stress Management and Mental Resilience

As we navigate the complexities of daily life, stress management and mental resilience are crucial for maintaining optimal brain health. While stress might seem like an inevitable part of life, it's empowering to know that there are practical ways to reduce its cognitive impact. By embracing regular techniques such as mindfulness and emotional regulation, we can effectively enhance our mental resilience, allowing us to bounce back stronger from life's challenges. Building these habits not only calms the mind but also fortifies it against future stressors. It's about cultivating a mental toolkit filled with personalized strategies that bolster emotional fortitude, ensuring that we don't just survive but thrive in the face of adversity. Building mental resilience is a dynamic process, one that equips us with the inner strength to adapt and grow continuously, fostering not only improved mental health but also enriched cognitive performance.

Techniques for Reducing Cognitive Stress

Life's pressures can really pile up, can't they? When your mind is juggling a hundred thoughts at once, cognitive stress is often the not-so- pleasant result. But here's the thing: stress doesn't have to be overwhelming. You can manage it effectively with the right techniques. Let's dive into some practical strategies for taming cognitive stress so you can thrive mentally.

First up, let's talk about breaking down tasks. The brain can feel like an overstuffed suitcase when you try to tackle everything at once. Breaking big tasks into smaller, more manageable chunks relieves that sense of overwhelm. Use a "to-do" list, but don't just write down huge tasks; go a step further and break them into subtasks. That way, every checkmark you make is a mini-celebration, giving your brain a small dose of satisfaction and reducing stress bit by bit.

Next, consider the magic of time management. Think about dedicating specific blocks of time to tackle various activities. The Pomodoro Technique, where you focus on a task for a set period (say, 25 minutes) and then take a short break, can enhance concentration and reduce procrastination. It also gives your mind periodic rest, which is crucial for reducing cognitive load.

Let's not underestimate the power of physical activity. A brisk walk or a short workout session can be a real game-changer for mental clarity.

Exercise increases blood flow to the brain, which helps you think more clearly and handle stress better. Anything that gets your body moving stands to combat that mental fatigue you feel after staring at your screen for hours on end.

Breathing techniques also deserve a mention. Maybe you've felt your mind racing during a stressful meeting or when you've got to meet a tight deadline. Techniques like diaphragmatic breathing or even a few minutes of mindful deep breaths can slow that racing mind down, reducing anxiety and bringing about a calming effect almost instantly.

Ever heard of progressive muscle relaxation? This technique involves tensing and then slowly releasing different muscle groups in your body. It acts like a reset button for your stressed-out mind. By shifting focus to physical sensations, this practice helps you disconnect from mental stress and fosters a deep sense of relaxation.

Journaling is another avenue worth exploring. It doesn't have to be a well-composed essay. Just get those thoughts and worries out on paper. This act of expression can provide clarity and help organize your thoughts. When you see your concerns written down, they often seem less daunting, bringing about effective stress relief.

Social support is a significant buffer against cognitive stress. A chat with a friend or family member can do wonders. Opening up about what's on your mind can lead to insights you hadn't considered. Plus, knowing you're not alone in your experiences can ease stress and improve your mental resilience.

A less obvious but powerful technique involves setting boundaries. In today's hyper-connected world, it's tempting to be constantly available, but this can lead to burnout. Learn to say no, and create some "me-time" where you can recharge. Set specific times to check your emails or messages, ensuring you have uninterrupted periods to focus on your tasks.

We can't talk about reducing cognitive stress without mentioning mindfulness and meditation, two approaches gaining popularity for good reason. Spending just a few minutes in meditation each day can ground you, centering your thoughts and reducing stress. Mindfulness allows you to focus on the present moment, which is a powerful deterrent to getting lost in stress-inducing spirals of "what if" thinking.

Nutrition plays a role too, more than you might think. The foods you consume affect your brain's stress response. Incorporating nutrient-rich foods, particularly those that boost brain health, can be a subtle yet effective way to help manage cognitive stress. Omega-3 fatty acids, antioxidants, and vitamins like B-complex are all worth considering.

Lastly, cultivating a positive mindset can significantly impact how you respond to cognitive stress. Embracing a growth mindset, where challenges are seen as opportunities to learn rather than obstacles, can liberate your mind from stress. Positive affirmations and gratitude practices can also shift perspective, helping you focus on what's going right rather than solely on the stressors.

So, tackle stress with these techniques in your toolkit. With a proactive approach, reducing cognitive stress becomes less an uphill struggle and more an integrated part of a healthy, mindful lifestyle. Remember, it's not about eliminating stress altogether—because life will always throw curveballs—but about building resilience and equipping yourself with strategies to handle stress effectively.

Building Emotional Resilience

Life throws curveballs at us all the time. Whether it's missing a flight, a job loss, or a global pandemic, challenges are inevitable. But what's important is how we handle these stressors and bounce back—or better yet, bounce forward. This is where emotional resilience comes in. It's the psychological muscle that helps us endure adversity and emerge stronger. And like any muscle, it can be developed and strengthened over time.

Imagine emotional resilience as the buffer that absorbs life's shocks. It's akin to physical fitness but for your mind. Just as regular exercise can enhance your body's capacity to endure physical stress, cultivating emotional resilience equips you to handle psychological stress. It's not about dodging the punches—it's about being able to take them, learn from them, and keep going.

Start Myth Self-Awareness: Developing emotional resilience begins with understanding yourself. Self-awareness is your first tool in the toolbox. It involves reflecting on how you react to stress and why you feel certain emotions in specific situations. What are your triggers? Which coping mechanisms do you usually resort to? Journaling can be incredibly helpful here—it's not just putting pen to paper but laying down a blueprint of your emotional landscape.

Next, build a positive self-identity. Confidence in your ability to handle challenges bolsters resilience. This doesn't mean you have to be overly optimistic all the time. In fact, healthy doses of realism can prevent disappointment. But believing in your capacity to overcome difficulties is crucial. Think of it as putting faith in your future self's resources and adaptability.

Social Connections Matter: Humans are inherently social beings. Our connections with others can either be a source of stress or a source of support, depending on how we manage them. Ask yourself: who are your anchors? Fostering healthy, supportive relationships can act as a protective factor against stress. These relationships are not just buffers—they're also lifelines, offering perspective and insights, which help you navigate tough times.

Conversely, recognize and manage the relationships that drain your emotional energy. Setting boundaries isn't selfish; it's necessary for mental resilience. Remember, you can't pour from an empty cup. Make sure you're surrounding yourself with people who fill you with positivity and encourage growth.

Mindfulness and Acceptance: While some stress management techniques focus on changing the external situations, emotional resilience often involves an inward turn. Mindfulness practices like meditation or controlled breathing help anchor us in the present. They cultivate an accepting attitude towards life's ups and downs. When we stop fighting the current and flow with it, strong emotions lose their power to destabilize us.

It's essential to understand that acceptance doesn't mean resignation to negative circumstances. Instead, it's about recognizing and acknowledging your emotions without judgment. This can be incredibly empowering.

You're telling yourself it's okay to feel the way you do—an affirmation that's necessary for emotional healing and growth.

Embrace Change and Adaptability: Change is the only constant, as the old saying goes, yet it's one of the most potent stressors. Here lies a paradox: while we're hardwired to preserve stability, evolution has endowed us with remarkable adaptability. Building emotional resilience involves nurturing this adaptability. Embrace changes as opportunities rather than threats. This simple shift in perspective can significantly enhance your ability to cope with stress.

What if things don't go as planned? That's perfectly fine. Sometimes a detour can lead to the most beautiful destination. Flexibility is an essential component of resilience. Try to view uncertainty as an open canvas, allowing you to paint your own path as you go.

Resilient Mindset: Fostering a resilient mindset is akin to planting a garden. You must nurture it consistently, pulling out weeds of negative thinking and sowing seeds of positivity and hope. Reframe setbacks not as failures but as stepping stones. This might sound cliche, but it works.

Cognitive reframing alters your perception, which in turn impacts your emotions and behavior.

Incorporate gratitude practices in your routine. Instead of focusing on what's going wrong, take stock of what's going right. Gratitude isn't just a feel-good exercise; it shifts your focus from stressors to things you appreciate. Over time, this shift can rewire your brain to be more optimistic and adaptive.

Self-Care as a Foundation: Finally, never underestimate the power of self-care in building resilience. Emotional resilience and physical health are closely linked. Ensure you're getting adequate sleep, nutritious food, and regular exercise. After all, a healthy body can nurture a resilient mind.

Spend time doing activities that recharge you. Participate in hobbies, take time off when needed, and carve out moments for relaxation and fun.

Self-care legitimizes your need for time and space, helping you manage life's challenges more effectively. Remember, taking care of yourself isn't a luxury—it's a necessity for maintaining emotional resilience.

Building emotional resilience doesn't happen overnight. It's a continuous process, much like a journey filled with different landscapes and experiences. Each step you take towards it is a step towards a better, more fortified version of yourself. Embrace the journey, cherish the learning, and watch as you build an unshakeable foundation of emotional resilience.

Chapter 7

Mastering Focus and Concentration

As we dive into mastering focus and concentration, let's explore how transforming your mental discipline can unlock unparalleled cognitive potential. When you harness the art of focus, distractions don't stand a chance. It all begins by implementing small, intentional changes—like setting clear goals and minimizing interruptions—that snowball into substantial improvements in your attention span. Regular mental breaks, mindfulness practices, and structuring your environment for success can elevate your ability to concentrate. When you commit to these techniques, you'll notice that not only do you increase productivity, but you also enhance your overall cognitive resilience. It's not just about working harder; it's about training your mind to work smarter, laying the groundwork for tackling life's challenges with unwavering clarity and purpose.

Techniques to Improve Attention Span

In a world brimming with distractions, honing our ability to concentrate seems both critical and elusive. From the constant ping of notifications to the myriad of digital channels vying for our attention, it can be challenging to maintain focus. Yet, strengthening our attention span is not only possible but essential for mastering focus and concentration.

Developing this skill can significantly enhance cognitive performance and improve overall mental resilience.

One of the most effective techniques to bolster attention span is practicing **mindfulness meditation**. By dedicating time to focus on the present moment without judgment, meditation helps individuals build a robust attention span. Research has shown that mindfulness practice increases gray matter in the brain regions involved with attention and self- regulation. Start with just a few minutes each day, simply focusing on your breath. Gradually increase the duration as you become more comfortable with the practice.

Another technique to consider is the **Pomodoro Technique**. This time management method encourages working in blocks of time, typically around 25 minutes, followed by a short break. By structuring work periods in this way, the brain learns to focus intensely for those intervals, improving attention and reducing mental fatigue over time. The key to success with the Pomodoro Technique is consistency—once it becomes a habit, the ability to concentrate will increase naturally.

Have you noticed the profound impact of staying physically active? Regular exercise is a powerful tool for enhancing cognitive functions, including attention span. *Exercise stimulates the release of neurotransmitters such as dopamine and norepinephrine, which play a crucial role in focus and attention.* Particularly, aerobic exercises like running or cycling have been shown to boost brain health, supporting sustained concentration. Incorporate at least 30 minutes of physical activity into your daily routine to maximize these benefits.

Fostering a clutter-free environment is another valuable technique for sharpening focus. The human brain is wired to react to visual stimuli, and a messy workspace can easily become a source of distraction. Simplify your surroundings by removing unnecessary items, and organize your workspace to enhance efficiency. This physical decluttering can mirror mental clarity, creating a conducive environment for better concentration.

In addition to physical organization, digital decluttering is equally important. As our lives become increasingly digitized, managing online distractions is crucial for maintaining focus. Consider using apps that block social media or limit exposure to distracting websites during work periods. By controlling digital temptations, you can protect your attention span and channel your energies into more productive pursuits.

Another strategy to improve attention is practicing the art of **single-tasking**. While multitasking might seem like an efficient way to tackle multiple tasks, it can lead to fragmented attention and stress. Instead, focus on completing one task at a time. This approach fosters deeper engagement with the task at hand, encouraging a steady and directed flow of concentration. Over time, your ability to maintain attention on a single task will strengthen.

There's also a deep connection between nutrition and attention span. Consuming a diet rich in omega-3 fatty acids, antioxidants, and essential vitamins can positively impact cognitive function. Foods like salmon, nuts, berries, and leafy greens are not only good for overall health but also improve brain function, which supports a longer attention span.

Hydration plays a role as well; even mild dehydration can impair cognitive abilities. So, remember to drink enough water throughout the day.

Consider implementing **scheduled breaks** into your working routine. Surprisingly, taking regular breaks can enhance focus by preventing mental fatigue and burnout. Whether it's a brief five-minute pause to stretch or a longer break to recharge, stepping away from your tasks can reset your mental state and drive. These breaks should allow you to step outside or engage in a non-screen activity to fully benefit from the interruption.

Furthermore, prioritize sleep. A well-rested mind is capable of maintaining focus for extended periods. Ensuring you get adequate rest each night is crucial for cognitive revitalization and the enhancement of your attention span. Establish a consistent sleep schedule, and create a restful environment to encourage quality sleep.

Lastly, encourage a mindset of continuous curiosity and learning. Engaging with novel experiences or tackling challenging problems stimulates the brain, keeping it agile and capable of sustained focus. By pushing your cognitive boundaries, you're constantly training your brain to adapt and expand its attention capacities.

By systematically adopting these techniques, you'll likely notice a marked improvement in your attention span. Such enhancements can lead to a more productive and fulfilling life. Mastering focus and concentration isn't just about tuning out distractions—it's about creating an optimal balance of mental clarity, environment, and routine. So, take these steps boldly, knowing each new habit formed is a stride towards a sharper, more resilient mind.

Overcoming Distractions

Let's face it; distractions are everywhere. Whether it's the notifications pinging on your phone, the constant barrage of emails, or unexpected interruptions, staying focused can feel like an uphill battle. However, mastering focus and concentration requires you to become a master at overcoming distractions. It's not just about blocking out noise, but also about training your brain to manage and prioritize stimuli effectively.

One powerful strategy for overcoming distractions is setting clear and intentional goals. When you know exactly what you aim to achieve, whether it's a small task or a long-term project, you're more inclined to maintain your attention on it. Use techniques such as the SMART criteria—ensuring goals are Specific, Measurable, Achievable, Relevant, and Time-bound—to fine-tune your focus. This allows you to create a clear roadmap of what needs to be done, which naturally minimizes the space for distractions to creep in.

Developing a routine can serve as an anchor against the winds of distraction. Establishing specific times for different tasks creates a pattern your brain can follow. This automaticity reduces the cognitive load of deciding what to do next and allows your mind to flow more freely, concentrating better on the task at hand. A consistent routine also easily identifies distractions for what they are—deviations from your intended path.

In the digital age, technology often acts as both a facilitator of productivity and a major source of distraction. It's crucial to harness technology wisely. This might mean setting boundaries, such as specific times for checking emails or social media, and sticking to these boundaries rigorously. Utilize apps and tools designed to block unwanted content or notifications, enhancing your ability to concentrate on what's important.

Some distractions are internal rather than external. Our minds often wander to thoughts unrelated to the task at hand. Incorporating mindfulness practices can be a game-changer. Techniques such as mindful breathing or short meditation sessions train your brain to recognize when it's drifting and gently bring it back to the focal point. It's about cultivating a state of awareness where you're conscious of distractions the moment they arise and can choose to redirect your focus.

An often overlooked factor in combating distractions is the environment around you. Your physical workspace can either promote a distraction-free zone or become a breeding ground for interruptions. Keep your environment tidy and organized. Have all the tools and resources you need within arm's reach, thus minimizing the need to get up and seek them. A well-lit, quiet, and ergonomically designed space enhances concentration by reducing physical discomfort that might otherwise divert your attention.

Sound can be a potent interrupter, but it can also be used strategically to minimize other distractions. Consider utilizing white noise or instrumental music to mask disruptive background sounds. This acts as an audio shield, allowing your cognitive faculties to focus solely on the task at hand. Experiment with different soundscapes to find what elevates your concentration levels best.

You can't underestimate the power of breaks. It might seem counterintuitive, but taking regular, short breaks actually enhances focus by preventing burnout and mental fatigue. Techniques like the Pomodoro Technique—where you work intently for 25 minutes and then take a 5- minute break—leverage cognitive rest to refresh and refocus your mind, readying it for the next bout of productivity.

Physical movement is another ally against distractions. Integrating some form of exercise into your daily schedule helps to reset your mental state and elevate your focus. A simple stretch or walk can be enough to release built-up tension and energize your brain, providing a fresh perspective once you return to your task.

Remember, focus is not a finite resource. It's a skill that can be honed and developed over time. Every small victory in overcoming distractions builds your concentration muscle, allowing it to naturally flex and strengthen without conscious effort.

By learning to identify your primary distractions, both internal and external, you can employ a variety of strategies to mitigate their impact. Each of these strategies serves a purpose—whether it's setting boundaries or optimizing your environment. The key is experimentation and adaptation. Find which tactics align best with your tasks and personal tendencies, and you'll go a long way in mastering focus and concentration.

Chapter 8

Memory Enhancement Techniques

Moving forward into memory enhancement techniques, we delve into ways to sharpen recall and bolster retention. Memory isn't just a passive receiver of experiences, but an active participant in processing and retaining information. Engaging in regular practice and reinforcement methods can transform your memory into an agile, reliable ally in the quest for knowledge. Attentive repetition and varied recall routines are key; they work like mental workouts, strengthening neural pathways and ensuring information sticks. Techniques such as visualization create vivid mental connections, making details easier to remember. Similarly, mnemonic devices convert abstract data into familiar patterns, facilitating quicker retrieval. Embrace these methods and you'll find your memory not only retains more but does so with surprising ease, unlocking doors to profound cognitive potential.

Memory Retention Strategies

Memory retention might feel elusive at times, but it's something within our reach when we understand how our brain works. You ever noticed how a certain smell can take you back to a childhood memory? That's your brain at work, pulling from its vast network of associations.

Memory retention strategies tap into these connections, enhancing our ability to recall information when we need it most.

Think of your brain as a muscle—it gets stronger with use. To boost memory retention, the cognitive load should be manageable, much like lifting weights at the gym. You wouldn't jump from tiny dumbbells to heavyweights overnight. Just as with physical strength training, memory can be strengthened through progressive challenges. This means pushing the boundaries of your memory capacity with incremental challenges, reinforcing those neural pathways each step of the way.

Association is a powerful tool for memory retention. Our brains are inherently wired to link new information to what's already lurking in our memory banks. Imagine that you're trying to remember a new person's name you just met at a party. The name itself might slip away, but if you associate it with something familiar—a similar-sounding object or a detail about the person—you're giving your brain an anchor to hold onto. This method, known as the *peg-word system* or *method of loci*, transforms abstract information into something tangible and relatable, enhancing recall.

Repetition undeniably plays a vital role. Ever heard of "muscle memory"? It's more than just a catchy phrase; it applies just as well to brain memory.

Frequent exposure to information strengthens the connections between neurons, making retrieval more automatic over time. Techniques such as spaced repetition, where learning is spread out over increasing intervals, optimize memory retention. It's like revisiting an old path repeatedly until it becomes instinctive, a shortcut in the dense forest of your brain's neuronal connections.

Moreover, storytelling is a fantastic vehicle for data storage in our brains. Narratives provide context and emotional engagement, which engrains information beyond rote memorization. When facts are woven into a compelling story, they're more likely to stick around. Educational systems often take advantage of this by weaving lessons into stories, making them memorable and engaging through relatable characters and plots.

Nutrition can't be ignored when discussing memory retention. The foods we consume can significantly impact how well our brain functions and its ability to hold onto memories. Omega-3 fatty acids are like brain food— literally feeding your brain the essential nutrients it needs to build cell membranes in the neurons that manage memory. While we're here, don't forget about antioxidants; they help protect your brain from oxidative stress, letting your neurons thrive.

Sleep shouldn't be underestimated either. While you're in dreamland, your brain is busy consolidating memories—flipping through the day's events, examining them, and stashing them where they belong. Without adequate rest, this critical process is disrupted. So, the next time you're tempted to burn the midnight oil, remember that a well-rested mind is a more efficient one, especially in memory consolidation and retention.

Then, there's the role of learning styles. People's brains are wired differently, which means a one-size-fits-all approach to memory retention doesn't exist. Whether you're a visual learner who benefits from diagrams and color codes, or an auditory learner who thrives off talking things out and listening to lectures, honing in on your preferred learning style can transform your memory abilities. Remember, it's all about leveraging your strengths to enhance memory retention.

Memory retention also benefits greatly from focusing on the moment and reducing external distractions. This is where mindfulness techniques shine. By sharpening our focus, we strengthen our attention span and improve memory retention. Concentration can grow, alongside our ability to retain new information, when we make a conscious effort to engage fully with the task at hand.

So, we've painted a broad picture of strategies that can enhance memory retention. By engaging with these strategies, you'll not only remember more but also access recollections with greater ease. Remember, your brain is a muscle—treat it kindly, nourish it well, and challenge it regularly, and it will repay you in kind with a sharper memory and an enriched life experience.

Practice and Reinforcement Methods

Memory isn't just a solitary skill; it's a work in progress, shaped and polished through consistent practice. By adopting effective practice and reinforcement methods, anyone can boost their memory capabilities significantly. Think of your memory like a muscle. Regular exercise and the right techniques can make it stronger. But how do we effectively practice memory enhancement?

Repetition stands as a tried-and-true foundation for memory retention. It's not just about mindlessly repeating information, but about engaging in deliberate practice. Think of a musician rehearsing their scales or an athlete perfecting their form. In memory practice, spaced repetition emerges as a powerful technique. Instead of cramming, this method involves reviewing information at strategic intervals, allowing your brain to encode and strengthen the memory pathways.

Beyond basic repetition, visualization offers a creative approach to reinforcement. When you tie information to vibrant, memorable images, it becomes easier to recall. This technique uses the brain's natural affinity for imagery to anchor abstract or complex information into something tangible. You've likely heard of the 'memory palace' technique, popularized by world memory champions. By mentally placing pieces of information in familiar, imaginary locations, you can improve recall with astonishing efficiency. It's about leveraging your mind's spatial and visual capabilities to organize and retrieve data better.

Active engagement with material is another cornerstone of memory practice. Simply put, practices like teaching someone else what you've learned or applying the information in real-world contexts solidify your understanding and recall. This is known as the 'Protégé Effect'. You might be surprised how much better you retain information when you're expected to share it with someone else.

Writing is another method that shouldn't be overlooked. Taking notes by hand activates different cognitive processes than typing. The deliberate movement involved in writing can help reinforce memory pathways. Moreover, summarizing information in your own words forces a deeper processing level, making the material stick with you longer.

Another lesser-known method is using mnemonic devices. Techniques like acronyms, rhymes, and chunks can significantly aid memorization. They provide a scaffold on which information naturally hangs.

Mnemonics transform bland data into something catchy and hard to forget. Imagine remembering a complex chemical formula because it sounds like a snappy jingle.

There's also the Pomodoro Technique, which serves dual purposes: it helps combat procrastination while reinforcing learning. By working in focused time blocks separated by breaks, this approach encourages sustained attention. The technique ensures that you're not only more productive but also more likely to recall material due to the focused practice involved.

Let's not forget technology's role in reinforcing memory practice. Apps like Anki or Quizlet leverage algorithms to perfect the spacing intervals needed for optimal retention. They're excellent tools for those learning languages or studying for exams, providing a personalized repetition schedule that's hard to replicate manually.

One fascinating aspect of memory practice is the role of emotions. When we emotionally engage with what we're trying to learn, retention improves. Think of how vividly you remember events filled with happiness, excitement, or even fear. When practicing memory techniques, find ways to emotionally connect with the material. Whether through personal stories or just a passionate interest in the topic, emotion can be pivotal.

The practice doesn't only have to occur in isolation. Group learning or study sessions can be highly beneficial. Discussions allow for different perspectives and corrections where necessary. These interactions not only reinforce information but also introduce a social dynamic that can make learning more engaging and less daunting.

Contextual learning is another innovative method to enhance memory retention. By associating information with specific settings or circumstances, you can improve recall. For example, studying biology in a park can evoke memories linked to a more natural environment, aligning theoretical knowledge with real-world context.

The rhythm of practice should be consistent and integrate daily routines. Integrating memory exercises into your daily life, like trying to recall your grocery list or reciting a poem during a walk, turns memory practice into a seamless part of living. This regular engagement ensures that memory enhancement isn't an isolated task but an ongoing endeavor woven into the fabric of day-to-day experiences.

Finally, reflection is crucial. Regularly reflecting on what you've learned consolidates memories and identifies areas that need more focus.

Reflective practices, like journaling or reviewing summaries, serve as a feedback loop, reinforcing what you've learned while highlighting gaps in knowledge.

Incorporating these techniques into everyday life might seem challenging at first. But like any good habit, once established, these practices become second nature. The investment you make today in reinforcing your memory will pay dividends in the form of a sharper, more agile mind in the days to come. Legacy isn't just about what you leave behind; part of it lies in the wisdom you acquire, retain, and pass on through a life well-lived and well-remembered.

Chapter 9

The Power of Lifelong Learning

Embracing lifelong learning is like unlocking a boundless treasure trove of potential within ourselves. It's not just about picking up new skills or earning additional credentials—it's about cultivating an ever-curious mindset that can morph into a powerful tool for cognitive enhancement. By consistently challenging our brain with fresh ideas and experiences, we nurture its elasticity and vitality, promoting mental agility that can adapt even to the most complex of life's puzzles. Picture lifelong learning as a vibrant garden where each new experience plants a seed of potential, which with nurturing attention, grows into a rich canopy of knowledge.

Moreover, this journey of perpetual education can fortify emotional resilience, making us better equipped to tackle life's ups and downs with grace and innovation. So, let's dive headfirst into the satisfying quest of continuous learning, knowing that every new chapter we absorb not only enriches our minds but sets the stage for a lifetime of growth and reinvention.

Benefits of Continued Education

In today's rapidly evolving world, the allure of lifelong learning can't be overstated. Continued education is like that secret sauce, and it's not just about keeping up with the latest trends; it's about enhancing your brain's vitality and opening doors you never knew existed. When you engage in ongoing education, you're inviting your brain to dance in a vibrant, intellectual symphony.

Let's consider the power of stimulation. When you learn something new, your brain creates and strengthens neural connections, making it more adaptable and resilient. This process is backed by the concept of neuroplasticity, which highlights the brain's incredible ability to reorganize itself by forming new connections. Continued education serves as an intense workout for your brain, similar to lifting weights that build physical muscles.

But it's not all science and brain waves; there's a personal aspect to it too. Learning keeps you humble and grounded. It reminds you that there's always more to discover, that you're never quite the master of everything. This mindset fosters a sense of curiosity and wonder, traits that are vital in maintaining a youthful spirit regardless of one's age.

Moreover, when you engage in continued education, you're not just gaining knowledge—you're enhancing your cognitive reserve. This reserve acts as a buffer against cognitive decline, potentially reducing the risk of age-related diseases such as Alzheimer's. By keeping your brain actively engaged, you're essentially future-proofing your mental faculties. It's a long-term investment in your cognitive wealth.

Of course, continued education isn't just about formal settings like universities or classrooms. It can be as simple as picking up a new hobby, reading a book, or taking up a language. The key is to remain inquisitive and open-minded, seizing opportunities to learn in everyday situations.

With every new skill acquired, whether through pottery classes or understanding quantum physics, your brain continues to grow and adapt.

Furthermore, engaging in lifelong learning can significantly boost your confidence and self-esteem. There's something incredibly fulfilling about mastering a new skill or understanding a complex topic. It empowers you to tackle challenges with greater assurance, knowing that you possess the ability to learn and adapt.

Learning also enhances your ability to connect with others. When you're learning new things, you gain a wealth of conversation topics, making you a more engaging and versatile social partner. Sharing insights from a recent course, or discussing the intricacies of a new debate, not only enriches your life but also strengthens your social bonds.

It doesn't stop there. Continued education can improve your professional life too. In an ever-changing job market, skills can quickly become obsolete. By keeping your knowledge and skills up to date, you're ensuring that you'll stay relevant and adaptable. This commitment to learning can open doors to new career opportunities, promotions, or even the ability to switch fields altogether.

Consider this: many industries are now prioritizing soft skills such as teamwork, communication, and emotional intelligence. These skills can be honed through various educational channels and are invaluable in navigating modern workplaces. Thus, the benefits of continued education stretch far beyond just the acquisition of hard skills; they encompass the overall growth and adaptability of an individual.

And let's not forget about the sheer joy of learning. There's a unique thrill that comes from those "aha" moments, when everything clicks into place and a new layer of understanding emerges. This intrinsic reward is a powerful motivator, driving you to explore even further.

In light of all these advantages, the quest for knowledge becomes an enriching journey with myriad rewards. While some may view education as a destination with a finite endpoint, embracing it as a continuous, lifelong process allows for endless possibilities. By fostering a commitment to lifelong learning, you're ensuring that you're not only enhancing your cognitive health but also enriching your entire life's narrative.

If you're wondering where to start, consider identifying areas you're passionate about or subjects you've always been curious about. Whether it's diving into the world of astronomy or exploring the intricacies of classical literature, the key is to follow your curiosity. Remember, lifelong learning doesn't have to be overwhelming; it should be joyful and fulfilling.

So, why not unleash your inner student and explore the uncharted territories of your intellect? The benefits of continued education are as vast as they are profound, offering you both personal satisfaction and enhanced mental acuity. As you embark on this journey of lifelong learning, may you find not just knowledge, but a deeper connection to the world around you and to yourself.

Developing a Learning Plan

The journey of lifelong learning is a powerful one, perhaps more so than any of us recognize at first. It's the continuous, self-motivated pursuit of knowledge, and it shapes how we adapt to the world around us. But such a journey isn't something you just stumble into fully formed. It needs a roadmap—a learning plan that guides and structures this voyage of discovery.

Creating your personal learning plan is akin to setting the coordinates on a GPS. It helps you identify where you want to go and the best routes to get there. Start by asking yourself some key questions: What do I hope to learn? Why is this knowledge important to me? How will acquiring this knowledge impact my life? This introspective questioning provides clarity and sets the stage for meaningful learning.

Once you've pinned down your motivations and objectives, the next step is to break them into achievable goals. Sure, you might have a broad aspiration, like becoming proficient in a new language or understanding quantum physics, but these can feel overwhelming if not broken down.

Imagine each goal as a series of stepping stones; you need to hop from one to the next steadily, not leap across a chasm. This incremental approach not only keeps you focused but also allows for regular reassessment of your progress.

So, how do you go about breaking down these goals? Consider employing the SMART criteria—Specific, Measurable, Achievable, Relevant, and Time-bound. This methodology ensures that each part of your learning plan is clear and actionable, preventing the drift that comes with vague objectives.

The backbone of any effective learning plan is consistency. Regularity in learning not only reinforces retention but also builds a habit. Create a study schedule that aligns with your daily rhythm. Maybe you're a morning person and can allocate time after breakfast, or perhaps nighttime suits you better. The key is to find a window where you're most attentive and least distracted, transforming learning into a natural part of your day.

While consistency is crucial, flexibility is equally important. Life is unpredictable, and rigid plans might crumble under unexpected demands. Allow room for adjustments in your schedule without feeling like you've derailed. Remember, the goal is progress, not perfection.

Don't overlook the value of diverse learning resources. We're living in an era where knowledge is at our fingertips in myriad forms. Books, podcasts, online courses, webinars, and hands-on workshops each offer unique perspectives and ways of understanding. Mixing up these resources keeps the process dynamic and engaging, catering to various learning styles and interests.

Pairing your learning plan with technology can also be a game-changer. Apps and online platforms can simplify tracking your progress and managing your resources. They can offer personalized recommendations based on your progress and even connect you with like-minded learners or mentors who can offer support and insight.

It's also worthwhile to incorporate reflection phases into your learning plan. Take time to review what you've learned, how you've applied it, and where you wish to go next. Reflection not only consolidates new knowledge but can breathe new life into your learning process by highlighting areas of interest you might not have considered before.

Motivation can be fleeting, but commitment to your learning plan keeps you on track. Celebrate small victories, however minor they seem.

Reward yourself for hitting milestones, be it finishing a challenging book or finally understanding a complex concept. These positive reinforcements fortify your commitment and make the learning process enjoyable.

Additionally, keep an eye out for feedback opportunities. Whether it's through formal assessments or casual discussions with peers or mentors, feedback offers invaluable insights into your progression. It helps illuminate areas needing improvement that you might have overlooked in self-assessment.

Collaboration can enrich the learning experience significantly. Study groups, discussion forums, and collaborative projects present chances for shared insights and alternate viewpoints. Engaging with others not only deepens understanding but fosters a sense of community, making learning a collective voyage rather than a solitary pursuit.

When developing a learning plan, don't shy away from challenges. A bit of friction can ignite curiosity and spur deeper exploration. Challenging topics or subjects force you to stretch beyond your comfort zone, fostering growth and resilience. Embrace setbacks as learning opportunities—they're stepping stones towards mastering more complex challenges.

Finally, keep your learning journey aligned with a broader life vision or purpose. When you're learning plan is connected to larger personal or professional goals, it gains a deeper significance. This connection ensures that every step forward is not just towards knowledge acquisition but also towards personal fulfillment and contribution to your community or field.

In conclusion, developing a learning plan is an essential step in harnessing the power of lifelong learning. It transforms abstract ambitions into concrete steps and sustains motivation by providing direction and focus. With a thoughtful and flexible approach, your learning plan becomes a lifelong companion, leading you towards constant growth and self-discovery. So, craft your plan with care, and set forth on your path of endless learning and boundless possibilities.

Chapter 10

Mind-Brain Relationship:

Insights and Applications

Diving into the mind-brain relationship unveils a complex yet fascinating dynamic that shapes how we perceive and interact with the world. Imagine the brain as the hardware—a sophisticated, biological computer—while the mind serves as the software that generates thoughts, emotions, and experiences. When these elements mesh seamlessly, we achieve cognitive harmony, enhancing problem-solving skills and emotional balance. Yet, the disconnect between them often fuels stress and hampers personal productivity. By harnessing insights from this relationship, you can unleash practical applications in your daily life, such as embracing mindfulness to bridge gaps or utilizing neurofeedback to optimize brain function. This exploration not only enriches self-awareness but also empowers you to tailor strategies that boost mental agility and resilience, turning abstract concepts into everyday action for a healthier, more fulfilled existence.

Understanding the Mind-Brain Disconnect

Diving into the mind-brain disconnect, we find a fascinating puzzle that has intrigued philosophers and scientists for centuries. It's a concept that challenges our comprehension of self, consciousness, and the intricate web of interactions that define human experience. On one hand, we have the brain, a physical organ composed of neurons and synapses, which processes information like a complex machine. On the other hand, there's the mind—a non-physical entity responsible for thoughts, emotions, and consciousness. The disconnect emerges because these two entities, though interdependent, don't always communicate seamlessly.

Picture yourself in a moment of intense stress: your heart races, palms sweat, and your mind spins in a whirlwind of thoughts. While your brain is processing signals, your mind may perceive them differently, perhaps even exacerbating your anxiety with spiraling thoughts. Here, the mind-brain disconnect can lead to a disordered stress response, affecting your well-being. Understanding this disconnect is crucial for developing strategies that help harmonize mind and brain, fostering mental clarity and emotional resilience.

The mind-brain relationship can be compared to a symphony orchestra, where each instrument must play in harmony to create beautiful music. When one section falls out of tune, the disconnect becomes apparent. In a similar vein, when the mind and brain fail to synchronize, it can result in cognitive dissonance. This dissonance might manifest as disjointed thinking patterns, emotional struggles, or even physical symptoms. To bridge this gap, it's essential to delve into the mechanisms and influences that govern these distinct yet overlapping realms.

Cognitive behavioral therapy (CBT) is a practical approach that often tackles the mind-brain disconnect. By changing thought patterns, individuals can influence brain activity, highlighting the intimate link between mental exercises and neurophysiological changes. This approach underscores the notion that altering our mental landscape can shape, and even rewire, brain pathways—a testament to the impactful relationship between mind and brain.

Understanding the disconnect also calls for a look into neuroplasticity, the brain's remarkable ability to reorganize itself by forming new neural connections throughout life. While neuroplasticity provides the brain with the flexibility to learn and adapt, the mind's perceptions can either enhance or hinder this process. Positive thinking and mindfulness practices, for example, can encourage beneficial plastic changes, reinforcing the mind's influence on brain structure and function.

Another compelling aspect of the mind-brain disconnect is how perception shapes reality. Our brains take in vast amounts of sensory data, yet it's the mind that interprets this data, often filtered through the lens of past experiences, emotions, and beliefs. This filter can create biases or blind spots, illustrating that while the brain provides raw data, the mind interprets it, sometimes leading to misunderstandings and distorted realities.

Throughout history, scientists have sought to measure and bridge the mind-brain disconnect through various models. One of the more contemporary theories proposed is the Integrated Information Theory, which suggests that consciousness arises from the interconnections and complexities within the brain's networks. Although this theory offers insights, it also lays bare the inherent complexity in fully unifying the mind and brain—a challenge that continues to spur research and debate.

Moreover, the disconnect can play a significant role in psychological disorders. Conditions such as depression, anxiety, and schizophrenia often involve a dissonance between perceived reality and brain function, leading to symptoms that affect an individual's quality of life. Advances in psychopharmacology and psychotherapy aim to realign mind and brain, demonstrating a dynamic interplay where understanding the disconnect can drive therapeutic innovation.

Our lifestyle choices also markedly influence the mind-brain connection. Factors like diet, exercise, and sleep impact brain chemistry, yet the mind's interpretation of physical states can magnify or mitigate their effects. For instance, chronic sleep deprivation can impair brain function, but an anxious mind might further amplify cognitive deficits by fixating on sleeplessness's repercussions. Thus, managing lifestyle elements with mindful intention can promote harmony between mind and brain.

Spiritual and philosophical explorations further enrich our comprehension of the mind-brain disconnect. Many traditions speak of a dualistic nature, proposing that bridging the gap involves spiritual practices aimed at aligning body, mind, and soul. Meditation, prayer, and other introspective activities create pathways for deeper awareness, sometimes serving as conduits to reconcile mind and brain imbalances.

Applications in technology also present intriguing possibilities for addressing the mind-brain disconnect. From brain-computer interfaces to virtual reality, these innovations provide new avenues for exploring and potentially narrowing the gap. As technology evolves, it offers powerful tools to enhance, measure, and perhaps even synchronize mind-brain dynamics, opening a frontier where science meets an age-old quandary.

In conclusion, the mind-brain disconnect remains one of the most compelling areas in cognitive science and personal development. By understanding and embracing this divide, we edge closer to unlocking potential and achieving a state of mental and emotional equilibrium.

Whether through therapeutic techniques, lifestyle changes, or cutting-edge technology, bridging this disconnect holds the promise of heightened

Well-being and a deeper understanding of what it means to be truly human.

Ultimately, the pursuit of connecting mind and brain paves the way for innovations in how we enhance cognitive function and nurture our mental health. As we continue to explore this complex relationship, we open doors to new possibilities, encouraging a harmonious existence where thought, emotion, and physiology connect seamlessly in the symphony of human experience.

Applying Insights in Daily Life

Understanding the intricate connection between the mind and brain is a remarkable step toward harnessing the full potential of human thought and behavior. However, the true value of this knowledge emerges when we apply it in our daily lives. These insights aren't just for theoretical analysis; they're tools we can use to enhance our daily experiences and interactions. Here's how you can seamlessly integrate these insights into your everyday routine to improve mental and emotional well-being.

One of the most accessible ways to apply these insights is by cultivating an awareness of your thoughts and emotions. Consider this: your thoughts shape how you perceive and react to the world around you. By becoming more mindful of your thought patterns, you can start recognizing negative cycles and work towards breaking them. Simple practices like

maintaining a gratitude journal or setting aside a few minutes for daily reflection can help transform your mindset over time.

Another potent application lies in the realm of decision-making. The relationship between mind and brain also influences how you make choices. By understanding how cognitive biases and emotional states impact judgment, you can develop strategies to make more balanced decisions. For instance, when facing a significant decision, try applying a structured approach that considers both logic and emotion.

Acknowledging how your current state of mind might sway your choices ensures you view options objectively.

The mind-brain relationship offers profound insights into stress management as well. Stress is an inevitable part of life, but how you respond to it can significantly affect your cognitive health. Recognizing the signals your brain sends when stressed, such as increased heart rate or scattered thoughts, empowers you to intervene promptly. Techniques like deep breathing, mindfulness meditation, or simply taking a brief walk can reset these stress signals, restoring your mental clarity and resilience.

Let's talk about the power of visualization techniques. Athletes and successful individuals often talk about envisioning success before they achieve it. This isn't mere wishful thinking. By visualizing desired outcomes, you engage your brain circuits and prime them for action. The process creates a mental blueprint, enhancing your focus and motivation. Whether preparing for a presentation or tackling a new challenge, envisioning your desired result can significantly boost your confidence and performance.

Habits are another critical component of applying mind-brain insights daily. Developing constructive habits can pave the way for sustained mental and physical health. The key is understanding how habits form and how they can be reprogrammed. It's a gradual process where small changes lead to significant impacts over time. Start with simple routines, like allocating fixed times for exercise or reading, and see how these deliberate practices influence your mindset and productivity.

Building interpersonal relationships is an area where these insights show substantial benefits. Social interactions aren't just about exchange of pleasantries; they deeply influence brain health. By fostering empathy and active listening, you can enhance these connections, making them more meaningful and rewarding. Understanding others' perspectives and emotions not only enriches your relationships but also helps you develop emotional intelligence, a crucial aspect of personal growth.

Another practical application is in fostering creativity. The mind-brain relationship suggests that a relaxed and open mental state can lead to innovative thinking. Encourage creativity by allowing yourself time to daydream or engage in activities outside your usual routine. This freedom from structured thinking allows your brain to make new connections, inspiring fresh ideas and solutions.

Your environment also plays a significant role in applying these insights. A cluttered space often leads to a cluttered mind. Creating a brain-friendly environment that embraces natural light, soothing colors, and plants can enhance your cognitive function and mood. Each element in your surroundings can either contribute to mental clarity or detract from it, so it's crucial to tailor your environment to support optimal brain health.

Finally, consider the role of continuous learning. Lifelong learning is one of the most effective ways to keep your mind engaged and healthy.

Whether it's picking up a new hobby, learning a language, or exploring new subjects, continuous learning challenges your brain, fostering neuroplasticity and cognitive vitality. Make learning a part of your daily routine with podcasts, online courses, or even casual reading sessions that broaden your horizons and stimulate your mind.

Applying these insights into your daily life doesn't require drastic changes. It's the small, consistent steps that lead to significant transformations. By being mindful of how the mind-brain relationship affects various aspects of your life, you hold the key to unlocking a more balanced, productive, and fulfilling existence. Each insight you apply builds upon the last, creating a sturdy foundation for your mental and emotional well-being. Embrace the journey, and let these insights guide you toward a more enriched and enlightened life experience.

Chapter 11

Creativity and Brain Function

Exploring the vibrant connection between creativity and brain function offers an intriguing glimpse into how our minds can innovate and inspire. Creativity isn't just about artistry—it's a complex cognitive skill that taps into multiple brain regions, lighting up neural pathways that often lie dormant. When we delve into our creative potential, we're essentially engaging our default mode network, fostering a harmonious dance between imagination and analytical thinking. This synergy not only enhances our solution-finding capabilities but also nurtures resilience in problem-solving. To encourage innovative thinking, indulge in activities that challenge conventional patterns, like sketching out-of-the-box ideas or brainstorming wildly imaginative scenarios. Each stroke of creativity reshapes our cognitive landscape, making our brains more adaptable, agile, and ready to meet the demands of tomorrow. Embrace it, for in creativity, we unlock the doors to limitless possibilities.

Unlocking Creative Potential

Creativity isn't just the domain of artists and musicians. It's a multifaceted aspect of cognition that enhances problem-solving, encourages innovation, and even supports mental health. The brain, a labyrinth of neurons, synapses, and untapped potential, holds the key to creativity.

Understanding how to unlock this potential can enrich your life in ways that go beyond merely creating art.

At the heart of unlocking creative potential is the idea that creativity can be developed and enhanced. It's not just a natural gift but a skill that can be honed through various strategies and mindsets. Much like neuroplasticity, the brain's ability to reorganize and form new neural connections, creativity thrives on openness and adaptability. When we engage with new ideas, environments, and challenges, we're essentially stretching our creative muscles.

One effective way to boost creativity is through the practice of divergent thinking. Divergent thinking is about generating multiple ideas and solutions rather than seeking a single, correct answer. It's the driving force behind brainstorming, free writing, and other exercises that push boundaries. In contrast to convergent thinking, which narrows down options to find the best solution, divergent thinking promotes exploration and experimentation, crucial for creativity.

If you've ever had a brilliant idea while taking a shower or walking in the park, you've experienced what's known as the incubation effect. This is the process of stepping away from a problem or creative project to allow your subconscious to continue working on it. When we let our minds wander, we often stumble upon unexpected insights and innovative ideas.

Environments play a significant role in creative potential as well. A cluttered or unappealing workspace can stifle creativity, while a well-organized space can stimulate it. Colors, light, and even background music can influence how creative or motivated we feel. Consider what ambiance works best for you and design your creative space accordingly. Personalizing your environment can create a sanctuary where creativity flourishes.

Mindfulness and meditation, although often associated with relaxation, also have a profound impact on creative thinking. These practices enhance focus and cultivate a sense of calm, clearing mental clutter. When the mind is uncluttered, it's more capable of making unique connections, thus enhancing creativity. Daily meditation, even for a few minutes, can lead to greater overall creative output.

Creativity is deeply linked with taking risks and embracing failure. Fear of failure often blocks creative expression, but understanding that mistakes are part of the process can be liberating. Each error or misstep is an opportunity to learn and grow. Embrace failure as a stepping stone on the path to innovation.

Collaboration is another powerful force in unlocking creative potential. When individuals come together, each person brings a unique set of skills and perspectives. This diversity can lead to creative breakthroughs that might not have been possible in isolation. Working with others also introduces accountability and shared enthusiasm, which can drive projects to completion.

It's also important to engage with varied disciplines and fields of study. When we step outside our primary areas of expertise, we expose ourselves to new perspectives and ideas. This cross-pollination of knowledge can spark creativity in surprising ways. Whether it's reading a novel outside your usual genre or attending a lecture in a different discipline, expanding your horizons fuels creativity.

Digital tools can be both a boon and a bane to creativity. On one hand, they offer vast resources and platforms for expression. On the other hand, excessive digital consumption and multitasking can diminish focus and creativity. Finding a balance is key. Use digital platforms wisely, leveraging them as tools for inspiration and collaboration while being mindful of screen time.

Another surprising enhancer of creativity is a healthy dose of daydreaming. Allowing the mind to drift can lead to unexpected connections and ideas. It turns out that a wandering mind isn't necessarily unproductive; instead, it can be ripe ground for creative insight. Give yourself permission to take mental breaks and see where your thoughts lead you.

Ultimately, unlocking creative potential involves a combination of internal and external factors. It's about cultivating the right mindset, creating an inspiring environment, and nurturing an openness to new experiences. By doing so, you can tap into the creative power that lies within you, enriching both your personal and professional life.

In summary, creativity is an innate potential waiting to be unleashed. From divergent thinking and collaboration to mindfulness and mindful digital usage, numerous strategies can nurture this ability. Embracing a growth mindset and erasing the fear of failure pave the way for innovation.

Unlock your creative potential, and you'll find a path to personal growth, problem-solving, and joy that you never knew existed.

Encouraging Innovative Thinking

When it comes to sparking new ideas and fostering innovation, the connection between creativity and brain function is paramount. Our brains are dynamic organs, always ready to form new connections and pathways. While creativity might feel mysterious, it's largely about harnessing these brain functions to generate different ways of thinking. Encouraging innovative thinking isn't merely about random bursts of insight; it's a process that can be nurtured and developed with intention.

Innovation often begins with curiosity. It might seem simple, but asking questions—and encouraging others to do the same—is a first step toward discovering new perspectives. By questioning assumptions and exploring alternatives, we not only expand our own thinking but invite others into a space where new ideas can flourish. This isn't just about asking the big questions either; sometimes, it's as simple as wondering about the 'why' behind everyday occurrences. This habit not only enhances our understanding of the present but also opens up avenues for future exploration.

The environment plays a significant role in fostering innovation. A supportive, stimulating environment that is rich in sensory inputs—colors, sounds, textures—can lead to a surge in creative thought. Spaces that encourage collaboration and free communication enable the free exchange of ideas, which is fundamental to innovation. When individuals feel safe to express unconventional thoughts, they are more likely to propose novel solutions. The brain thrives in these conditions, as it is continuously seeking to link disparate elements into cohesive, ground-breaking ideas.

Moreover, embracing risk and failure is crucial for innovative thinking. People often talk about learning from failure, yet the fear of failing can be a significant barrier to creativity. Successful innovators are usually not afraid to test uncharted waters, even if it means failing along the way.

Each failure is a stepping stone towards a more refined and effective solution. Embracing experiments—even those that don't turn out as Planned —pushes us closer to groundbreaking discoveries. In this broader context, failure isn't just acceptable but necessary for progress.

Innovative thinking is closely linked to lateral thinking, where solving problems requires an indirect and creative approach. This conscious shift from linear to lateral thinking often leads to more substantial breakthroughs. By encouraging the exploration of ideas that are not immediately related to the problem at hand, we enable a free flow of thoughts and insights that might be overlooked through traditional logic. Cultivating habits of lateral thinking involves engaging in activities that challenge the brain to think differently—such as puzzles, games, or exploring arts and culture.

Critical to innovation is the practice of mindfulness. Meditation and mindfulness can improve attention, focus, and ultimately, creativity. When our minds are clear and focused, we create more space for innovative thinking. Mindfulness practices allow us to tap into a deeper well of creativity by quieting the constant chatter of the mind, thereby unlocking access to fresh insights and ideas.

Cross-disciplinary learning is another pathway to innovation. By integrating knowledge and methodologies from diverse fields, we produce novel solutions that might not arise from a single discipline. Encouraging collaboration between different areas of expertise, whether in art, science, technology, or humanities, often results in creative solutions that challenge existing norms. This is partly because our brains enjoy creating new connections, and the mix of disparate ideas can lead to 'Eureka' moments.

Building an innovative mindset also requires fostering intrinsic motivation. When the drive to create and innovate comes from within, it is more sustainable and effective. Encouraging people to pursue their passions and interests satisfies their curiosity while fueling their desire to create. A key element here is autonomy—allowing individuals the freedom to explore and create without constraints or excessive control.

This intrinsic motivation serves as a catalyst for sustained innovative thinking and problem-solving. Encouraging innovative thinking is also about promoting diversity in thought and experience. Different perspectives can inspire unique ideas, and blending these perspectives can lead to innovative breakthroughs.

Encouraging diverse teams, whether through varied cultural backgrounds, experiences, or methodologies, can lead to more comprehensive and far-reaching creative outcomes. Such diversity enriches the creative process, broadening the array of ideas and solutions available.

Finally, creating a habit of reflection is essential to innovation. After an event or project, taking the time to reflect on what went well and what could be improved provides valuable insights for future endeavours.

Reflection allows us to learn from experience, understand our internal processes, and apply this understanding to nurture future innovation. This practice of delving into detailed introspection, understanding, and learning can deeply enhance creative output.

Understanding and nurturing these elements of brain function and creativity can not only lead to personal growth and development but can also empower us to contribute meaningfully to the world around us. By cultivating an environment and mindset conducive to innovative thinking, we pave the way for advances and breakthroughs that might have once seemed unreachable. In essence, innovation isn't a reserved domain for a few; it is reachable and available to anyone willing to engage with these dynamic brain processes.

Chapter 12

The Aging Brain: Myths and Facts

Aging gracefully doesn't just apply to our bodies, but to our brains too. Yet, myths often cloud our understanding of what actually happens up there as the years tick by. The idea that cognitive decline is inevitable is an exaggeration, though changes certainly happen. Our brain retains the ability to adapt even as it ages, thanks to neuroplasticity. What's crucial is distinguishing fact from fiction about these changes, enabling us to combat aging with the right strategies. Regular mental exercises, a balanced diet, and an active lifestyle can all play pivotal roles in maintaining brain health. By debunking myths and embracing evidence- based approaches, we arm ourselves with the tools needed to sustain cognitive vitality and even continue growing mentally. Emphasizing the right practices can make aging an opportunity for wisdom, not just loss.

Understanding Cognitive Decline

Cognitive decline—it's a phrase that can stir worry as we age, touching nerves about our mental sharpness slipping away. But understanding it involves sorting through a mix of fears, facts, and intriguing biological mysteries. While it's a natural part of aging, the extent and impact vary greatly among individuals. Yet, dispelling myths and embracing informed perspectives can empower us to approach brain health proactively.

The aging process isn't merely about losses and decline. Think of it as a shift in priorities within your brain. This perspective allows us to see that while some cognitive abilities might slow, others like wisdom and emotional insight often blossom. So, what's happening beneath the surface in our minds as the years tick by?

To put it simply, cognitive decline refers to the gradual decrease in cognitive functions such as memory, attention, and the speed of thought processes. It's important to note: not all decline signifies disease. Age-related changes are typical, akin to gaining physical experiences like wrinkles or grey hair. What becomes crucial is distinguishing between normal aging and conditions like mild cognitive impairment (MCI) or dementia which require clinical attention.

Several key changes take place in the brain as we age. Neurons, the brain's signal carriers, start to shrink and lose some connections. Additionally, blood flow in the brain may decrease, meaning less oxygen and nutrients reach our critical thinking centers. The brain also starts to produce fewer chemicals responsible for sending messages between neurons. Sounds daunting, right? However, it's not all downhill.

Neuroplasticity, the brain's ability to reorganize itself by forming new neural connections, plays a heroic role in aging. It's how your brain can adapt and compensate for these age-related changes. Learning new skills, challenging the mind with puzzles, or simply engaging in stimulating conversations can encourage this plasticity, effectively curbing cognitive decline.

Despite the broad consensus on these physiological changes, the degree and speed of cognitive decline differ widely due to various factors such as genetics, lifestyle choices, and pre-existing health conditions. For instance, individuals with a higher educational background tend to show less cognitive decline. But why is that? It's believed their brains have built up a "cognitive reserve," an extra capacity to endure damage longer before showing signs of slowing down.

Adopting a healthy lifestyle, including balanced nutrition and regular physical activities, isn't just about keeping fit—it's crucial for brain health. A consistent routine that involves mental exercises, proper rest, and stress management can stave off early cognitive decline. Sure, it's easier said than done, but every step forward counts. Engaging with your community, learning new languages, or even picking up an instrument—these are all avenues to strengthen your cognitive reserve.

Moreover, appreciating cognitive decline includes acknowledging the psychological side of aging. This process isn't merely about clinical symptoms; it's about attitudes and interpretive frameworks toward growing older. Our perceptions wield significant power over our experiences. Viewing aging as a natural, manageable phase rather than an inevitable decline can foster resilience and motivation to seek out constructive lifestyle adjustments.

Of course, intervention is sometimes necessary. Identifying the signs of pathological cognitive decline early, such as significant memory loss or confusion impacting daily life, allows for timely medical consultation and planning. Technologies in brain imaging and advances in neuroscience provide powerful tools to detect and assess these issues at earlier stages than ever before.

In navigating the complexities of cognitive decline, maintaining an open dialogue with healthcare providers is vital. Leveraging their insights and tests assures a factual understanding and aids in planning interventions or ongoing support tailored to individual needs. Recommendations could involve cognitive therapies, medications, or lifestyle modifications to mitigate progression rates.

Culturally, cognitive decline has worn a cloak of stigma, contributing to stereotypes and misunderstandings about aging populations. Yet, good public awareness and informed consciousness can foster supportive environments where everyone feels encouraged to cultivate brain-healthy habits throughout life.

Emphasizing the collective effort to redefine cognitive health, organizations and communities are investing resources in awareness campaigns, educational programs, and supportive services. Their aim is empowering individuals with knowledge, reassurance, and actionable strategies to manage their cognitive well-being effectively.

Understanding cognitive decline should bring more empathy and awareness of the rich complexities entailed in aging. Remember, the essence of this journey isn't about eradicating decline but learning how to navigate and enrich the voyage toward continued growth and fulfillment.

Strategies to Prevent Aging Effects

As we delve into the complex world of the aging brain, it's crucial to distinguish fact from fiction. Many believe that cognitive decline is an unavoidable part of getting older, yet that's not the whole truth. While some changes in brain function are natural with age, there are numerous strategies to mitigate these effects and even enhance cognitive vitality as years go by. Let's explore effective methods to keep our brains thriving.

First and foremost, physical exercise is a powerhouse for brain health. Not only does regular physical activity improve mood and energy levels, but it also triggers neurochemical changes that bolster brain function.

Exercise increases blood flow, delivering oxygen and nutrients to the brain, and promotes the creation of new neurons, a process known as neurogenesis. Whether it's a brisk walk, a cycling session, or a dance class, finding an activity that brings joy ensures it's a sustainable part of one's lifestyle.

In the realm of nutrition, a brain-supportive diet is equally transformative. The Mediterranean diet, rich in vegetables, fruits, whole grains, nuts, and fish, has been linked to a lower risk of cognitive decline. Omega-3 fatty acids, prevalent in oily fish like salmon and sardines, are particularly beneficial for maintaining brain health. They help reduce inflammation and are crucial for neural function. Additionally, leafy greens, berries, and nuts are packed with antioxidants that fight oxidative stress, a key player in brain aging.

Equally important is staying mentally active. Just as physical exercise keeps muscles robust, cognitive activities challenge the brain, strengthening neuronal connections. Engaging in puzzles, learning a new language, or even volunteering for a complex task are excellent ways to remain mentally spry. Lifelong learning shouldn't be underestimated, as it fosters neural adaptability, often referred to as neuroplasticity, which allows the brain to reorganize itself in response to new experiences.

The power of social connections in maintaining cognitive health is often understated. Social interactions encourage emotional regulation and provide intellectual engagement. This doesn't mean one needs a bustling social calendar; even a small circle of meaningful interactions can stimulate cognitive function and ward off feelings of isolation or depression, both of which are detrimental to brain health.

Adequate sleep is another cornerstone of a healthy, aging brain. It might feel challenging to prioritize sleep amidst life's demands, yet its restoration effects are indispensable. Good sleep cycles consolidate memories, remove toxic waste products, and keep mood and stress levels in check. Establishing a relaxing bedtime routine and ensuring a peaceful sleeping environment can be game-changers for superior sleep quality.

Your brain's resilience against aging is also bolstered by managing stress effectively. Chronic stress reduces the size of the brain areas involved in memory, such as the hippocampus, and impairs cognitive function.

Techniques like meditation, yoga, and deep breathing exercises reduce cortisol levels, enhancing brain health and emotional well-being. These practices don't only cultivate calmness; they fortify the brain's capacity to handle stressors with grace.

Incorporating mindfulness into daily life keeps us grounded in the present, slowing down the whirlwind of worries that often accompanies aging. Mindfulness meditation sharpens attention and has been shown to improve memory, mood, and overall cognitive flexibility. Even a few minutes a day focusing on breath or sensations can have profound long-term impacts.

The narrative wouldn't be complete without acknowledging the revolutionary role of genetics and epigenetics in brain aging. While genetics lay the blueprint, lifestyle choices can influence how genes are expressed. This epigenetic process means you're never entirely at the mercy of your genes but can actively control aspects of your cognitive health through lifestyle adjustments.

Engaging in recreational activities that spark joy and stimulate creativity—such as painting, music, or writing—offer more than just pleasure. They encourage innovative thinking and offer protection against the monotony that can accelerate cognitive decline. By fostering creativity, you're not only enriching your immediate experience but also providing your brain with the mental dexterity it craves.

The conscious design of a supportive environment also influences cognitive health. De-cluttering spaces, ensuring ample natural light, and incorporating elements of nature can markedly affect focus and mental clarity. These adjustments encourage a brain-friendly habitat that not only looks pleasant but supports cognitive function over the long haul.

Trying to balance all these strategies might seem daunting at first, yet approaching them incrementally can turn aspirations into actionable habits. Starting small, perhaps with five-minute breathing exercises or a morning walk, can integrate these changes seamlessly into your daily routine. Each step, although small, culminates in a significant impact over time.

The aging brain is not just a vessel of diminishing capacity but one of lifelong growth and adaptation. By harnessing these strategies, you can proactively shape a future where your brain isn't merely surviving but thriving, filled with richness, resilience, and vitality.

Chapter 13

Social Interaction and Brain Health

Engaging with others isn't just about swapping stories and laughter; it's a vital component of cognitive wellness. Social interaction plays a remarkable role in keeping our brains sharp, enhancing mental agility, and even warding off neurological decline. When we communicate, listen, and empathize, our brains light up with activity, creating new connections and reinforcing existing pathways. Think of it as exercise for your mind, but with the added benefit of human connection. Building meaningful relationships provides emotional support, which further cultivates resilience and wellbeing. So, whether it's a heartfelt chat over coffee or a lively debate, these social exchanges are more than just pastime—they're a cornerstone of brain health that motivates and inspires us to maintain rich and fulfilling lives. Prioritize them, and you might just find yourself feeling more focused, spirited, and mentally alive.

Importance of Socializing for Cognitive Function

Socializing isn't just about the fun and laughter it brings into our lives; it's a cornerstone of mental agility and overall brain health. Human beings are inherently social creatures, and our brains are wired to interact with others. The mental gymnastics involved in daily conversations, negotiating meanings, and building relationships enrich our cognitive abilities. These interactions stimulate our brain, fostering a sense of belonging while also enhancing our problem-solving skills.

Interestingly, engaging in social activities can be just as challenging for your neurons as playing a game of Sudoku or learning a new language. This challenge comes from the need to process complex information swiftly, respond appropriately, and adjust to the social dynamics at play. Every smile, frown, and word exchanged in conversation adds layers of meaning that our brain must decode. In doing so, brain regions responsible for emotional regulation, language processing, and memory are all simultaneously activated.

Consider the cognitive demands of a simple social interaction. When you're talking to someone, you're not only processing their words but also taking note of their body language and responding in a way that matches the context. This complex coordination tasks our brain with maintaining and accessing a broad range of information, a process that is crucial for sharpening our memory and enhancing executive function.

So why does socializing hold such power over cognitive function? For one, it combats loneliness, which has been shown to have detrimental effects on brain health. Loneliness doesn't just feel uncomfortable—it can lead to cognitive decline and is associated with conditions like dementia and Alzheimer's disease. The potential for these outcomes underscores why maintaining social ties is vital at all stages of life.

Moreover, engaging in social activities can significantly boost your mental health. Positive interactions release neurotransmitters such as dopamine and serotonin, chemicals known for improving mood and concentration. This can create a ripple effect—when you're in a good mood, and your concentration is sharp, you're more likely to engage in activities that further enhance your brain function. It's a cycle that can ultimately protect against cognitive aging.

Think back to a time when you participated in a group activity or team sport. The ebb and flow of teamwork require strategic planning, quick decisions, and effective communication. These elements don't just contribute to the success of the activity but also serve to exercise the brain's capacity for attention, coordination, and multitasking. Such activities demonstrate that socializing in structured environments like clubs or teams can provide significant mental workouts.

For those who may feel socially anxious or introverted, digital advancements offer a comforting solution. Virtual platforms and online communities can also serve as amazing outlets for social interaction, catering to various interests and allowing for connections across distances. The digital world opens doors to forums and chat rooms where people can engage with others on topics they are passionate about, without the anxiety of face-to-face interaction.

Connection through socializing serves as a protective barrier against cognitive decline. The simple act of a conversation involves encoding, storage, and retrieval processes that are vital for memory and learning. Studies have shown that individuals who maintain strong social networks are less likely to experience memory loss, even displaying better cognitive function than those who are isolated.

What's the takeaway here? Make social interaction a staple in your mental fitness routine. Whether it's a phone call, group walks, or a hobby club, any form of engaging with others can contribute to mental sharpness. How you choose to socialize can be as unique as you are—it's about making it a consistent part of your life. Approach it like any other essential practice for brain health, such as regular exercise or balanced nutrition.

The diversity that comes with mixing different personalities, opinions, and experiences also promotes cognitive flexibility. When you are exposed to differing viewpoints, your brain gets a good workout evaluating and assimilating information, thereby boosting your critical thinking abilities. These challenges and experiences from social interactions offer one of the richest environments for cognitive rehearsal and growth.

Undoubtedly, the precise impact of socializing on brain health can vary from person to person. However, it's clear that it offers substantial benefits across various cognitive dimensions, piqueing curiosity and fueling intellectual vitality. Incorporate social interactions more consciously into your efforts for cognitive enhancement, and you'll likely find yourself not only with a sharper mind but also a more enriched life overall.

Building Meaningful Relationships

In today's fast-paced world, the ability to forge and maintain meaningful relationships is more crucial than ever, not just for emotional well-being but for brain health, too. Social interaction is a cornerstone of cognitive vitality. When we share experiences, emotions, and thoughts with others, we engage various parts of our brain that stimulate neural pathways and enhance neuroplasticity. But what makes a relationship meaningful, and why should we focus on building it?

Strong and meaningful relationships often go beyond surface-level interactions. They involve a deep connection that requires effort, understanding, and empathy. This process is akin to exercising a muscle; the more we work on our connections, the stronger and more resilient they become. By prioritizing quality over quantity, we allow ourselves to build trust and mutual respect, leading to more fulfilling and rewarding interactions.

Studies have shown that people who maintain close relationships with friends, family, and community members tend to have better cognitive health as they age. These interactions provide mental stimulation, encouraging cognitive engagement and problem-solving. When we interact with others in a meaningful way, we challenge ourselves to think differently, reflect upon our beliefs, and adapt to new perspectives—key components that contribute to cognitive longevity.

Loneliness and social isolation can have severe consequences on brain health. They aren't just emotional states that diminish emotional wellness; they can lead to cognitive decline. When people feel disconnected, their brains miss out on the vital cognitive exercises that social interactions provide. This lack of engagement can lead to stress and even accelerate the onset of conditions like dementia. Therefore, it's crucial to actively seek out and nourish the connections that prevent these negative effects.

One of the key elements in building meaningful relationships is effective communication. Engaging in open and honest dialogue with those around us fosters understanding and strengthens bonds. The act of sharing thoughts, listening earnestly, and responding empathetically keeps our brains active and alert. These interactions stimulate the release of oxytocin, a hormone that reduces stress, promotes well-being, and enhances social memory.

Flexibility in our interactions also plays a vital role. No relationship is perfect, and adaptability helps navigate through challenging times. By addressing conflicts constructively and forgiving mistakes, we maintain healthier connections that contribute to a stable and supportive social network. This adaptability also encourages cognitive flexibility, an essential trait for strong problem-solving skills and creativity.

Moreover, participating in shared activities can forge stronger connections and create lasting memories. Whether it's volunteering, joining clubs, or simply enjoying leisure activities together, these shared experiences build rapport and encourage teamwork. They introduce novel ideas and situations, prompting the brain to think outside the box, learn, and grow.

It's important to recognize that building meaningful relationships doesn't happen overnight. It's a continuous process of nurturing and growth.

Relationships need attention and care, much like any other aspect of our health. This might involve having regular check-ins with loved ones, prioritizing face-to-face interactions over digital communications, and acknowledging and appreciating the unique qualities that each person brings to the table.

While technology offers unprecedented ways to connect, it's essential to ensure these connections retain depth and substance. A quick text message or social media like cannot replace a heartfelt conversation or a shared laughter. Thus, consider using technology as a bridge rather than a destination. Use it to plan face-to-face gatherings or to maintain relationships with loved ones who are far away.

Incorporating gratitude into our social interactions can also make a significant difference. Expressing appreciation and recognizing the efforts of others reinforces positive behavior and strengthens bonds. This simple act can lead to a chain reaction of goodwill and mutual respect, further deepening the connections that hold significant cognitive and emotional benefits.

Thus, a meaningful relationship is not just a source of joy and happiness but a powerful tool for maintaining robust brain health. By being proactive in cultivating and nurturing our social connections, we unlock the potential for a more engaged, fulfilled, and cognitively enriched life. As we weave these intricate networks of care and trust, our brains do the same, mapping out resilient neural connections that stand the test of time. In this way, we're not only enhancing our personal lives but also contributing positively to our cognitive wellness.

Chapter 14

Technological Interactions and Brain Health

As we find ourselves in an era where technology is interwoven into the fabric of our daily lives, its influence on brain health is both profound and multifaceted. We engage with screens more than ever—through smartphones, tablets, and computers—each interaction contributing to a complex tapestry of cognitive impacts. While technology can be a double- edged sword, offering tools for enhanced cognitive abilities and potentially overwhelming our sensory inputs, it's crucial to strike a balance. Understanding the pros and cons of screen time allows us to harness technology in a way that supports our brain health without letting it control our lives. Incorporating regular digital detoxes is one way to regain this balance, giving our brains the much-needed breaks to rejuvenate. These intentional pauses not only foster mental clarity but also nurture our intrinsic abilities for deep thinking and creativity. By navigating this digital age with mindfulness, we can ensure our relationship with technology remains conducive to brain health and overall well-being.

Pros and Cons of Screen Time

In today's digital age, screens are everywhere—from smartphones to tablets, laptops to televisions. They have become integral to our daily lives, providing access to a world of information and entertainment at our fingertips. But as we embrace this digital culture, it's essential to weigh the benefits and drawbacks of screen time, particularly when it comes to brain health. Is it harming or helping us? Let's explore this dynamic and fascinating topic.

On the pro side, screens offer unparalleled access to information and learning resources. In this era of technological evolution, knowledge isn't confined to libraries or classrooms. With the internet, individuals can take online courses, attend webinars, and participate in virtual discussions across the globe. This digital access can stimulate the brain, encourage lifelong learning, and enhance cognitive skills.

Moreover, technology has revolutionized the way we communicate. Video calls and social media have made it easier to stay connected with family and friends, which is crucial for maintaining strong social ties. As we know from our previous discussions on social interaction and brain health, these connections can reduce feelings of isolation, support emotional well-being, and bolster cognitive function.

Let's not forget the entertainment value of screens. Engaging in games and recreational activities on digital devices can bring joy and relaxation, which are beneficial for reducing stress and enhancing mood. Many games also challenge the brain, promoting strategic thinking and problem-solving skills. These activities can serve as a form of mental exercise, sharpening cognitive skills as we age.

However, on the flip side, excessive screen time has its downsides. Perhaps the most significant is its impact on sleep. We've highlighted the importance of quality sleep for cognitive performance in an earlier chapter, and screens can interfere with this. The blue light emitted from screens can disrupt the natural sleep cycle, leading to poor sleep quality, which in turn affects memory consolidation and focus.

Additionally, there's a risk of developing a sedentary lifestyle. With increased screen use, especially when it's a significant part of one's routine, physical activity levels can plummet. This lack of movement can have negative implications for brain health, as regular physical activity is vital for maintaining cognitive function and neuroplasticity.

Furthermore, overindulgence in screen time may lead to stress, anxiety, and even depression. The constant barrage of notifications and the pressure to keep up with information can be overwhelming. Many individuals find themselves glued to their devices, driven by a need for validation or fear of missing out (FOMO), which can be mentally exhausting.

There's also the concern about concentration and attention spans. With access to a limitless stream of content, the ability to focus on a single task without distraction can diminish. This multitasking culture can lead to more superficial cognitive processing, affecting the quality of attention and long-term retention of information.

Another significant drawback is the potential for digital addiction. This relates to the behavioral impact of constantly using devices, leading to compulsive connectivity. Such habits can dominate a person's life, affecting everything from work to personal relationships, and leading to an unhealthy dependence on digital devices.

Balancing screen time is crucial, and many find that setting limits is an effective strategy. Encouraging regular breaks, promoting offline activities, and establishing screen-free zones or hours in homes can be beneficial. Additionally, utilizing technology with a purpose rather than as a default activity can help regulate screen use and ensures it adds value to one's life.

One more thing: introducing mindfulness practices, which you've already explored, can be a fantastic way to counteract screen time's downsides. Being present and aware of how much time we spend on screens can prevent the mindless scrolling that often leads to negative outcomes.

It all comes down to a conscious approach to technology usage. By understanding and managing the pros and cons of screen time, we can make informed choices that enhance our brain health and overall well-being. It's about harnessing the benefits of digital interactions while remaining aware of their limitations, maintaining harmony between our tech-driven world and personal cognitive goals.

In summary, screen time presents both opportunities and challenges for brain health. When used mindfully, technology can be a powerful tool for learning and connection. But without balance, it can lead to cognitive disruptions, physical inactivity, and emotional stress. So, as we continue to embrace the digital age, let's strive for a healthy relationship with our screens, one that prioritizes our brain health and enhances our quality of life.

Digital Detox Techniques

In our hyper connected world, digital devices have become almost an extension of ourselves. It's no wonder that managing screen time is an ever-present concern for maintaining brain health. As we continue exploring the relationship between technology and our minds, learning how to perform a digital detox becomes crucial. It's not about cutting technology out altogether—it's about using it wisely and finding that elusive balance.

One powerful technique is setting specific "tech-free times" each day. Consider allocating the first hour after waking or the last hour before sleep as sacred times for quiet reflection or personal interaction without the interference of screens. This can help in resetting one's cognitive focus and allows for more genuine social interactions. Shifting these moments away from screens can reinvigorate the senses and often leads to improved sleep quality and mental clarity.

Another effective approach is to create physical spaces in your home or workplace marked as "no-tech zones." Designating places like the dining room, bedroom, or a cozy nook in your living room as digital-free can encourage face-to-face conversations and bolster deep thinking.

Psychologists suggest that associating certain spaces with relaxation or engagement, free from digital disturbances, reinforces patterns of mindfulness and presence.

For those who find themselves habitually reaching for their phones, app audits are a wise strategy. Scrutiny of the applications on your device to determine which ones really add value and which merely drain time is vital. Uninstalling or disabling non-essential apps can reduce digital noise, giving your brain the rest it deserves. Utilize focus modes or app limit features available on most smartphones, which can act as gentle reminders to take a break from the digital world.

If you're looking for a more structured approach, consider setting specific digital goals. This might involve scheduling "tech sabbaths" once a week, where you unplug completely and engage in offline activities like reading, hiking, or crafting. Having dedicated days away from screens allows the brain some respite, leading to heightened creativity and less stress. These intentional breaks from technology can be surprisingly refreshing, offering a renewed perspective and sense of calm.

Leveraging technology against itself is a clever tactic in your detox arsenal. There are numerous apps designed to track digital usage and promote healthier habits. Such tools analyze the time spent on devices and offer insights into usage patterns that might need re-evaluating. This feedback can be eye-opening and inspires more disciplined use of technology.

Social media, while a significant digital platform for connection, often contributes to cognitive overload. Practicing mindfulness in how you consume social media is another vital technique. Consider adopting methods such as limiting social media to certain times of the day or curating your feeds to follow only content that truly enhances your life. Mindful scrolling can reduce anxiety and foster a healthier digital interaction.

For the more adventurous, a complete digital detox retreat could be the answer. These are typically structured getaways that focus on no tech engagement, allowing participants to connect with nature or engage in activities that draw them away from their usual digital habits. Retreats often provide a comprehensive reset, offering a taste of life unanchored from a digital device, and give participants new tools to manage their digital habits upon returning to daily life.

Being proactive about managing our digital interactions often involves leveraging community and having accountability partners. Share your goals with friends or family who can support and join in on the digital detox journey. This can create a community bond over shared experiences, making the process less daunting and more enjoyable.

Implementing "batch processing" for communication can be surprisingly effective. Instead of allowing notifications to interrupt your day, designate specific times to check and respond to emails, messages, or social media. This practice not only minimizes distractions but can significantly enhance productivity and mental peace.

Finally, remember that the key to a successful digital detox lies in its gradual introduction and flexibility. It's crucial not to view it as a rigid rule but as fluid strategies that adapt to your needs. Customize your approach so it complements your life rather than creating added stress. With the right mindset, a digital detox becomes more about gaining rather than losing.

The success of these techniques isn't measured by how much time you can go without your phone, but rather by how enriched and balanced your life becomes as a result. As you navigate this path, your mind will thank you—rewards include heightened creativity, less anxiety, better sleep, and more meaningful connections in your non-digital world.

Chapter 15

The Role of Positivity in Cognitive Health

As we dive into the world of cognitive health, the importance of maintaining a positive mindset can't be overstated. Studies and anecdotes both tell us that positivity isn't just about feeling good—it's a transformative force that enhances brain function. Embracing optimism and cultivating a positive outlook can lead to increased mental resilience, better problem-solving skills, and even improved memory retention.

When you're positive, your brain focuses on possibilities rather than roadblocks, which can alleviate stress and promote overall cognitive wellness. Think of positivity as a workout for your brain, encouraging flexibility, strengthening neural connections, and boosting your ability to adapt to life's challenges. Shaping a mindset that sees the silver lining in every cloud doesn't just contribute to better cognitive health—it also lays the foundation for a fulfilling, vibrant life where your mind can thrive in harmony with your emotional and social well-being.

Positive Thinking and Mental Strength

In the realm of cognitive health, the impact of positive thinking and mental strength stands out as a significant contributor. Our thoughts not only color our mood and perception but also shape our brain structure over time. The power of positivity isn't just anecdotal; it's backed by science. When we weave positive thinking into our daily narrative, it influences the plasticity of our brains, enhancing cognitive function and resilience. It's akin to a mental workout that keeps our neural pathways robust and agile.

Exploring the connection between positive thinking and enhanced mental strength, consider that optimism isn't about ignoring life's hurdles. Rather, it's about approaching challenges with a constructive mindset. This disposition builds a foundation for resilience, helping you recover from setbacks more swiftly. By training your mind to lean towards the positive, you're also fortifying your mental resilience. It’s like laying down mental habits that bolster your ability to cope with stress and adversity efficiently.

Let's take a closer look at how positivity can strengthen your mental faculties. When consistently practicing positive thinking, your brain undergoes structural changes. For instance, studies have shown increased activity in the prefrontal cortex and hippocampus areas, which are linked to emotional regulation and memory. Consequently, you're not just feeling better mentally; you're enhancing parts of your brain responsible for crucial cognitive tasks like decision making and memory recall.

One effective approach to cultivating positivity is reframing negative thoughts. This doesn't mean pretending everything's perfect, but rather, shifting perspective to see opportunities within challenges. Recognizing your capacity to adapt and grow can be transformative. When you face a difficult task or an unexpected change, try to find any lesson or silver lining hidden within the situation. Over time, this practice of reframing will fortify your mental resolve and help create new, more positive neural connections.

Another aspect of positive thinking is its relationship with stress reduction. Being optimistic doesn't eliminate stress, but it buffers against its negative impacts. When facing stressors, those with a positive mindset tend to experience lower levels of cortisol, the stress hormone. This doesn't just feel good – it has tangible health benefits like improved immune function and reduced risk of chronic illnesses. So, by nurturing positivity, you're not just boosting your mood; you're improving your overall health outlook.

The role of gratitude in fostering positive thinking can't be overstated. Regularly practicing gratitude is like a workout for your mind. It directs your focus onto what's going well, fostering a profound sense of well-being. Keeping a gratitude journal, where you jot down a few things you're grateful for, is a simple yet powerful exercise. This practice can lead to increased positivity over time, and it lays down a neural foundation of abundance and resilience.

Mental strength is often misperceived as innate talent, but it's really a skill you can develop. Positive thinking acts as the cornerstone in building this skill set. Just as athletes practice consistently to sharpen their physical abilities, cultivating a positive mindset requires practice and commitment. Techniques like positive visualization can be a strong ally here.

Envisioning successful outcomes can prepare your mind for real-life success by creating a mental blueprint for achievement.

Social interactions also play a vital role in reinforcing positive thinking and mental strength. Engaging with friends, family, and communities that promote positivity can have a profound effect on your mindset.

Conversations filled with encouragement and support can help you maintain a constructive outlook on life's challenges. This social aspect not only strengthens emotional bonds but also creates a network of mutual support that can uplift everyone involved.

Even while positivity shapes mental strength, it's essential to acknowledge and validate negative emotions. They play a vital role in our psychological landscape, acting as signals that something might need attention or change. By understanding and addressing these feelings, you can approach them from a place of insight rather than denial. This balanced approach ensures mental health remains whole, resilient, and adaptive.

In closing, nurturing positive thinking and mental strength is an ongoing journey – a daily practice that enhances your cognitive health and overall well-being. It's about consciously choosing optimism and resilience, even when faced with challenges. By actively engaging in this mental cultivation, you'll not only meet life's ups and downs with a steady mindset, but you'll also create lasting positive change in your brain's architecture. And that, indeed, is a powerful testament to the human spirit's incredible capacity for growth and renewal.

Cultivating a Positive Mindset

Cultivating a positive mindset can feel like finding sunlight in a world often clouded by negativity. It doesn't mean ignoring life's challenges or pretending everything's perfect. Rather, it's about deliberately choosing to focus on solutions instead of dwelling on problems. Positivity acts like a balm for our minds, helping to soothe stress and foster resilience. By consistently working on maintaining an upbeat outlook, you can enhance your cognitive health and enrich your life experiences.

The influence of positive thinking on brain health is profound. Studies have shown that maintaining an optimistic attitude can not only reduce stress but can actually enhance your brain's problem-solving capabilities. When you're optimistic, your brain embraces creativity, enabling you to see beyond the immediate obstacles and imagine greater possibilities.

This kind of thinking is like a workout for your brain, promoting greater flexibility and resilience, much like how exercise tones muscles and boosts physical endurance.

One of the key steps to cultivating a positive mindset is self-awareness. Being aware of your thoughts, emotions, and reactions is crucial to understanding where negativity might be rooted. Self-awareness provides you with the clarity needed to make conscious efforts to shift your perspectives. For instance, instead of spiraling into frustration when faced with a challenging task, recognizing that frustration can be a trigger allows you to pause and reframe the situation—perhaps viewing it as an opportunity to learn something new or to strengthen a skill.

Cultivating gratitude is another powerful tool in fostering positivity. Gratitude isn't just about being thankful; it's about finding joy in the little things and appreciating the journey. Taking a few moments each day to jot down what you're thankful for can significantly elevate your mood and alter your brain's wiring to lean towards positivity. Simple reflections like these, even focusing on ordinary events like a sunny day or a friendly conversation, can amplify happiness and reduce the tendency to ruminate on the negatives.

Another strategy involves surrounding yourself with positive influences. This doesn't mean you need to cut off everyone in your life who's having a tough time. Instead, choose to engage with people who uplift you, inspire you, and encourage you to be your best. The energies and attitudes of others can profoundly impact your brain's chemistry. Positive interactions release oxytocin, the bonding hormone, which enhances feelings of trust and empathy, creating a supportive network that energizes and nurtures your cognitive wellness.

Practicing positive affirmations can be surprisingly effective, especially for boosting self-esteem and self-efficacy. Affirmations, when repeated consistently, help to rewire your brain, replacing doubt and insecurities with reassurance and confidence. Imagine starting each day with a simple statement: "I am capable and ready to tackle the challenges ahead." Over time, such affirmations can transform your mindset, subtly encouraging you to approach situations with a sense of empowerment and confidence.

It's important to note that maintaining positivity is not about suppressing negative emotions. Emotions like sadness, anger, and disappointment are natural and have their place in a balanced emotional life. The aim is to avoid getting stuck in these states. Allow yourself to feel and process these emotions, but also focus on transitioning back to a more balanced or positive outlook, recognizing that negative experiences often provide invaluable lessons and growth opportunities.

Mindfulness practices, such as meditation and deep breathing exercises, can also be instrumental in cultivating positivity. These practices encourage living in the present moment, which reduces anxieties tied to future uncertainties or past regrets. Through mindfulness, you learn to appreciate what is, not what could be or what might have been, bypassing the natural tendency of the mind to wander into negative territory.

At times, life can throw curveballs that make sustaining a positive mindset feel daunting. During these times, consider focusing on what's within your control. By honing in on manageable tasks or small steps forward, you maintain a sense of agency. Even on challenging days, achieving a small, positive goal can create a ripple effect, boosting your confidence and reinforcing the mindset that you're capable of overcoming difficulties.

Lastly, remember that cultivating a positive mindset is a journey, not a destination. Some days will be easier than others, and that's perfectly okay. Consistency is key. Over time, you'll find that your brain adapts to this new norm, creating neural pathways that favor positive thoughts and actions. In doing so, the positivity you cultivate today sows seeds for a resilient, agile mind ready to face the future with enthusiasm and courage.

Chapter 16

Understanding Brain Injuries and Recovery

The human brain's resilience is truly awe-inspiring, especially when it faces the monumental challenge of recovery from an injury. Brain injuries can range from mild concussions to severe traumatic impacts, each with its own path to recovery. What's incredible is how the brain, through its remarkable plasticity, can adapt and forge new pathways even after significant damage. Rehabilitation plays a critical role here, harnessing this adaptability through targeted therapies and exercises designed to restore functionality and independence. It's not just about healing—it's about tapping into the brain's innate ability to rebalance and innovate, often leading to unexpected breakthroughs in individual capabilities. Recovery might be a complex journey, riddled with obstacles, but the potential for regaining cognitive functions and even achieving newfound strengths is immense. Embracing patience, persistence, and focusing on incremental progress can empower individuals to overcome the challenges presented by brain injuries and look forward to a future of continual growth and adaptation.

Types of Brain Injuries

Brain injuries can be a daunting topic, steeped in medical jargon that often feels overwhelming. Yet, understanding them is crucial for anyone keen on brain health and cognitive enhancement. These injuries, quite diverse in nature, can impact our mental functions and the recovery journey we might embark upon. They are often classified based on the cause or the nature of the injury, which can range from traumatic to non-traumatic.

Let's dive into the different types of brain injuries with the aim to demystify and simplify this critical subject.

Traumatic Brain Injuries (TBI): Whenever we hear about brain injuries, TBIs are often the first to come to mind. These injuries result from an external force impacting the head, commonly seen in accidents, falls, or sports injuries. They can range significantly in severity, from a mild concussion that temporarily affects cognitive abilities to severe injuries leading to long-term complications. One hallmark of TBI is the potential for subtle or overt changes in thinking, sensation, language, or emotions. Treatment approaches are varied but usually involve a combination of medical interventions, rehabilitation therapies, and, importantly, time.

One of the most discussed outcomes of TBI is a concussion, a mild form of brain injury. Although it's labeled "mild" due to the absence of life-threatening symptoms, the effects can sometimes be quite debilitating.

Symptoms like headaches, confusion, and dizziness might linger long after the incident. Athletes are particularly at risk, and increasing awareness about safe practices and protective gear is crucial.

Coup-Contrecoup Injuries: This form of brain injury involves a dual process where the brain crashes into one side of the skull (the coup injury) and then rebounds to strike the opposite side (contrecoup). Such injuries tend to occur in severe car accidents or falls, where significant force is exerted. The double impact can cause bruising, bleeding, or swelling, leading to complications that require comprehensive treatment strategies.

Diffuse Axonal Injury (DAI): Rather than being caused by a direct blow, DAIs occur due to the brain stretching beyond its capacity. They're common in situations involving rapid acceleration or deceleration, like a vehicle collision or intense rotational forces. This stretching damages nerve pathways, disrupting communication between nerves and affecting various brain functions. DAIs can be particularly challenging because they may not always show clear symptoms initially but still lead to significant long-term cognitive and physical impairments.

Non-Traumatic Brain Injuries: Contrary to TBIs, non-traumatic brain injuries arise from internal causes. They include strokes, aneurysms, infections, or tumors, among others. Let's consider stroke, one of the more prevalent non-traumatic injuries, which occurs when the brain's blood supply is disrupted. This can result in cell death, causing permanent impairments. The road to recovery involves a blend of medication, rehabilitation, and lifestyle modifications.

Another notable form is *anoxic brain injury*, where the brain is deprived of oxygen for prolonged periods. Causes might include near-drowning incidents, heart attacks, or severe respiratory conditions. Oxygen is vital for brain cells, and even a brief shortage might lead to significant damage, reinforcing the need for rapid medical intervention to minimize damage.

Hypoxic Brain Injury: Similar yet distinct from anoxic injuries, hypoxic brain injuries occur when oxygen levels are below optimum but not entirely absent. For instance, exposure to high altitudes or carbon monoxide poisoning can cause such injuries, emphasizing the importance of environment and external conditions on brain health. The symptoms and recovery depend largely on the duration and severity of the oxygen shortage.

The variety in brain injuries extends to their symptoms, treatments, and recovery paths, underscoring the importance of personalized approaches in medical care. Brain injuries don't affect everyone the same way; they respect no boundaries of age, occupation, or background. The severity and impact can vary widely, manifesting in anything from mild cognitive challenges to severe disabilities.

Understanding the different types of brain injuries isn't just for medical professionals but for anyone invested in personal development and cognitive enhancement. Being aware means you can better support those around you who might be dealing with these challenges, as well as protect yourself proactively. Whether it's by advocating for better safety measures in sports or seeking immediate medical help after a hard knock to the head, awareness is our first line of defense.

For those on a recovery journey post-injury, the road might seem long, filled with physical therapy sessions, cognitive exercises, and an adjustment to new ways of navigating the world. Yet, it's crucial to remember that with the right support and interventions, recovery is not only possible but can also lead to profound personal growth and resilience. This is where the power of positive thinking, patience, and perseverance shines.

As you further delve into this subject, bear in mind that each brain injury is unique. Treating and recovering from these injuries often requires a tailored approach. Advances in neuroplasticity—the brain's incredible ability to heal and adapt—are offering fresh hope. While the journey can be arduous, it's also filled with opportunities for innovation and discovery. Let's continue to spread awareness, advocate for better safety, and support each other in creating environments that foster brain health and recovery.

Rehabilitation and Recovery Approaches

Rehabilitation and recovery from brain injuries require a combination of perseverance, precision, and personalized care. Understanding that each brain injury is as unique as the individual experiencing it is fundamental to developing effective strategies. Rehabilitation is not merely about regaining lost functions; it's a profound journey toward redefining abilities and embracing a new reality.

Central to recovery approaches is the incorporation of neuroplasticity principles. Our brains, despite profound injuries, possess the remarkable ability to adapt and reorganize. This adaptability offers hope and a pathway to regaining function and independence. Rehabilitation programs often incorporate targeted exercises that harness this inherent plasticity, creating new neural connections and strengthening existing ones.

One effective rehabilitation approach is cognitive rehabilitation therapy (CRT), designed to improve cognitive function through structured exercises. These exercises focus on enhancing memory, concentration, problem-solving, and critical thinking skills. CRT often involves repetitive drills and gradually increasing complexity to challenge the brain, encouraging growth and resilience.

Physical therapy plays a crucial role in recovery, particularly for those dealing with motor impairments post-injury. Therapists employ techniques that improve mobility, strength, and coordination, promoting the brain's ability to form new motor plans. The goal is to encourage independence and improve quality of life through enhanced physical capabilities.

Occupational therapy is another essential component, focusing on helping individuals regain the ability to perform daily tasks. This includes everything from personal grooming to using technology for communication. Occupational therapists work closely with patients to develop tailored strategies that accommodate their specific strengths and weaknesses, fostering a sense of achievement and autonomy.

Speech and language therapy addresses communication challenges arising from brain injuries. Therapists help individuals improve verbal and non-verbal communication skills, enabling better interaction with the world around them. This type of therapy often involves exercises to enhance articulation, comprehension, and social communication behaviors.

In some cases, psychological support is vital for addressing the emotional and behavioral changes that can accompany brain injuries.

Psychotherapists help individuals cope with feelings of frustration, anxiety, or depression, which are common responses to such life-altering events. By building emotional resilience, individuals can maintain a positive outlook, which is crucial for long-term recovery.

Community reintegration programs aim to help individuals transition back into their daily environments. These programs provide support in returning to school, work, or other social settings, emphasizing the importance of community support and inclusion. Social workers and rehabilitation specialists often facilitate these transitions, providing guidance and advocacy as needed.

Technological advancements have greatly enhanced rehabilitation strategies. From virtual reality to brain stimulation devices, technology offers innovative ways to engage brain plasticity and expedite recovery. For instance, virtual reality allows patients to practice real-world tasks in a safe environment, while brain stimulation devices can enhance learning processes during therapy sessions.

It's essential to acknowledge the role of caregivers in the rehabilitation process. They provide crucial support and encouragement, often acting as advocates for their loved ones' needs and progress. Caregivers must also be educated and involved in the rehabilitation journey, ensuring a collaborative approach that maximizes recovery outcomes.

A multidisciplinary team approach is often most effective, involving professionals across various specialties. Neurologists, psychologists, physical and occupational therapists, and speech-language pathologists all contribute their expertise to create a comprehensive, personalized recovery plan. This collaborative effort ensures that every aspect of the individual's well-being is addressed, promoting holistic recovery.

Setting realistic and patient-centered goals is a key aspect of rehabilitation. Celebrating small victories and making adjustments along the way helps maintain motivation and morale. Recovery journeys are inherently personal, and understanding that progress can be non-linear is crucial for both patients and caregivers.

Recovery is not just about physical and cognitive healing. It involves rebuilding identity, confidence, and self-worth. Encouraging individuals to pursue their interests and passions during rehabilitation can provide emotional fulfillment and a sense of purpose, accelerating overall recovery.

The journey to recovery after a brain injury is challenging but deeply rewarding. It requires patience, persistence, and the unwavering belief in the brain's ability to adapt and heal. By embracing the diverse approaches to rehabilitation, individuals can forge paths to recovery that are as unique as they are. Through structured support and innovative therapy, new chapters of life emerge, filled with hope, growth, and renewed potential.

Chapter 17

Brain Health Myths and Misconceptions

It seems like everywhere you turn, someone's touting a new 'fact' about brain health—some outdated, others just plain wrong. Let's cut through the noise. You'll often hear folks claim that brain cells can't regenerate, but that's just one of the myths we're here to debunk. Thanks to neuroplasticity, our brains are actually capable of forming new connections and even new cells throughout our lives. Or take the age-old belief that a decline in cognitive function is inevitable with age. Science shows there are plenty of strategies to keep our minds sharp well into our golden years. With this chapter, we're diving head-first into these myths, backed by solid, evidence-based facts that inform and inspire. So as we move forward, remember: just because something's repeated often doesn't make it true. A well-informed perspective is your most powerful tool for maintaining brain health and avoiding the pitfalls of half-truths.

Debunking Common Misbeliefs

The world of brain health is ripe with myths and misconceptions that often lead us astray. It's fascinating—and a tad bit bewildering—how some notions about the brain can become so entrenched in our minds that we consider them gospel truth. Yet, dispelling these myths is essential for anyone dedicated to truly enhancing their cognitive health. Your brain deserves better than to be shackled by outdated beliefs.

One popular myth is that we only use 10% of our brains. This idea, perpetuated by pop culture and movies, suggests that unlocking the rest of our brain's potential could grant us superhuman abilities. However, neuroscientists unanimously debunk this myth. Through advanced imaging techniques, we've seen that we use almost every part of our brain, even when we're asleep. Complex brain activities like memory, decision-making, and developing creativity engage multiple areas of the brain, simultaneously painting a picture that is far more vibrant and active than the 10% myth suggests.

Another common misbelief is that intelligence is solely based on genetics and cannot be changed. While it's true that your genetic makeup plays a role in shaping your cognitive profile, the environment—what you do, what you eat, how you live—has a significant influence too.

Neuroplasticity, the brain's remarkable ability to reorganize itself, enables us to improve our cognitive abilities regardless of age. Engaging in

Brain-stimulating activities, learning new skills, and maintaining an active lifestyle can stimulate brain growth and enhance cognitive function. This dynamic capability to adapt and evolve insightfully proves that we're more than the sum of our inherited traits.

People often believe that memory declines irreversibly with age. This fear leads many to accept memory lapses as an inevitable consequence of aging. However, this isn't entirely accurate. While some cognitive functions may slow with age, other areas, like vocabulary or wisdom, can remain stable or even improve. Engaging in memory enhancement techniques and maintaining a healthy lifestyle can significantly mitigate age-related memory decline. It's all about staying mentally active and challenging the brain regularly.

Stress is a normal part of life, but not all stress is bad for the brain. Contrary to the belief that stress always harms cognitive function, there's something known as "eustress"—positive stress that can enhance brain performance. For instance, a challenging work project can spark motivation and improve focus, acting as a natural catalyst for cognitive growth. The management of stress, rather than eliminating it entirely, is key to maintaining optimal cognitive health. Techniques like mindfulness and meditation are effective means of transforming negative stress into positive outcomes.

Many people assume that the brain capsizes permanently and cannot heal itself once injured. The narrative of irreversible brain damage is slowly being rewritten, thanks to research showing the brain's capacity for recovery. Neurorehabilitation strategies are now helping individuals regain functions post-injury, leveraging neuroplasticity to rewire and compensate for damaged areas. It should be noted that recovery isn't instantaneous or guaranteed, but the potential for the brain to heal itself fosters hope for countless recovering patients.

A misconception that often circulates is the belief that left-brained individuals are analytical while right-brained people are creative. This divide has become a cultural meme, but it oversimplifies how our brains operate. In reality, the brain is much more integrated. Both hemispheres work in tandem to facilitate a wide range of activities—from solving math problems to composing music. Creativity and analysis are products of a whole-brain process, transcending the simplistic left-right divide.

Another myth that hangs in the air is the idea that a bigger brain equates to greater intelligence. It's a notion that's been debunked over time. The size of one's brain doesn't correlate with intelligence levels; instead, it's the network of connections within the brain and how efficiently these connections function that determines cognitive prowess. It's not about having a larger brain; it's about having a better-connected one.

It's crucial to challenge the myth that saturated fat directly feeds your brain and leads to cognitive decline. While extreme consumption of unhealthy fats can negatively affect your brain and body, the brain actually needs a certain amount of healthy fats to function correctly. Foods rich in omega-3 fatty acids, such as avocados and nuts, support cognitive function. The balance here is crucial; moderation is key.

People often credit creativity to only the naturally gifted, but creativity, like many other traits, can be cultivated. Believing that creativity is unteachable restricts individuals from exploring their innovative capabilities. Engaging in creative exercises, brainstorming new ideas, and embracing unfamiliar concepts can all help boost creative thinking .

Everyone possesses a wellspring of creativity waiting to be tapped into; it's merely a question of practice and openness to experience.

Sleep is essential for brain health, yet another myth persists that you can "catch up" on lost sleep and negate its negative effects. The reality is more nuanced. While sleeping in after a rough week might feel restorative, it doesn't fully compensate for the cumulative impact of chronic sleep deprivation on your brain. Sleep routines and quality over quantity play a significant role in maintaining cognitive health and ensuring mental alertness.

Finally, let's tackle the myth that the brain stops developing at a certain age. The discovery of neurogenesis in adults challenges the belief that brain cell production halts in childhood. By continuously learning and staying active, you can encourage the growth of new neurons even in advanced age, underscoring the brain's lifelong capacity for regeneration and growth.

By debunking these myths and misconceptions, we open up a world of possibilities for improving brain health. It's a thrilling endeavor, guiding us to engage actively with our cognitive potential rather than being sidelined by incorrect beliefs. Embrace the knowledge and let go of the myths, for a healthier and more enlightened understanding of your brain's capabilities.

Evidence-Based Facts

We all want to get smarter, think faster, and boost our brainpower. But in our pursuit of brain health and cognitive enhancement, it's easy to fall for myths that don't hold up to scrutiny when examined through the lens of science. Let's cut through the misconceptions and focus on what evidence- based research has to say.

First off, there's the idea that popping supplements can instantly make you a genius. The market brims with so-called "smart drugs" and brain supplements that promise enhanced memory, clarity, and focus. While some nutrients are vital for cognitive function, like Omega-3 fatty acids and B-vitamins, most supplements lack substantial scientific backing.

Consuming them isn't a magical fix. A balanced diet rich in whole foods often meets the body's needs without requiring expensive pills.

Exercise is another misunderstood factor in brain health. The myth that only aerobic exercise is beneficial for cognitive function diminishes the role of strength training. Recent studies suggest lifting weights can significantly impact brain health, boosting neurogenesis and improving memory. Aerobic exercise remains crucial, but don't skip the weights assuming they're only for "bulking up." Each form of exercise has its unique advantages.

Another prevalent myth is the belief that brain games are the key to sustained mental agility. Popularized by apps promising to sharpen minds through daily exercises, these games improve performance in their specific tasks, but their effectiveness in enhancing overall cognitive function isn't well-supported by evidence. Real-world activities like learning a musical instrument or acquiring a new language provide broader cognitive benefits, engaging multiple brain areas rather than focusing on specific game-induced skills.

Many have heard that the adult brain is hardwired, incapable of change. Neuroplasticity, the brain's ability to reorganize itself by forming new neural connections, debunks this. Advanced imaging technologies and studies reveal that adults can indeed grow and adapt their brains, not just through new learning but also by changing their environment and experiences.

You've probably encountered claims of strict brain hemispheric dominance, where you're either "left-brained" (logical, analytical) or "right-brained" (creative, innovative). In reality, although certain functions are lateralized to one side, both hemispheres consistently work together. Tasks often require a blend of analytical and creative processes, making this myth an oversimplification of brain function.

Sleep is often sacrificed in our busy lives, with some myths claiming that high achievers thrive on minimal rest. However, scientific evidence highlights that sleep is indispensable for memory consolidation, emotional regulation, and cognitive performance. Sleep deprivation impairs decision-making and problem-solving abilities, underscoring the need for consistent, quality rest.

The myth that intelligence is entirely predetermined by genetics can be discouraging, but it overlooks the role of environmental influences and personal effort. While genetics do play a significant part, our environment and the choices we make can greatly impact our cognitive abilities. Lifelong learning and adopting a brain-healthy lifestyle encourage cognitive growth, challenging the notion of fixed intelligence.

Social interaction is sometimes underestimated in its importance for brain health. Loneliness and social isolation have negative implications for cognitive function, often being associated with a higher risk of cognitive decline. Evidence shows meaningful relationships and social networks support cognitive health by providing emotional support and mental stimulation. So, staying connected with others isn't just a nice-to-have; it's imperative for maintaining cognitive sharpness.

The rise of technology has also fueled misconceptions, particularly that screen time inherently damages our brains. While excessive use, especially without breaks, can lead to issues like eye strain and poor posture, focused and mindful utilization of technology can be beneficial. Tools can facilitate learning and communication, provided they're balanced with offline activities.

Finally, let's dispel the myth that positivity is just a soft science. Maintaining a positive mindset can indeed bolster brain health, with studies linking positive thinking to reduced stress levels, better problem-solving, and improved overall well-being. Cultivating positivity isn't about ignoring challenges, but adopting an approach grounded in resilience and adaptability.

In conclusion, understanding brain health requires distinguishing fact from fiction. Acting on science-based insights rather than myths equips us to make more informed choices about our cognitive well-being. By embracing these evidence-backed facts, we pave the way for healthier minds and more fulfilling lives.

Chapter 18

Future Directions in Brain Research

Peering into the future of brain research is like standing on the edge of a new frontier, ripe with transformative potential. With emerging technologies like advanced neuroimaging techniques and brain-computer interfaces, we're set to unravel the mysteries of the mind in ways previously unimagined. Imagine artificial intelligence aiding in mapping neural connections or personalized medicine tailoring cognitive solutions based on unique genetic profiles. We're on the brink of potential breakthroughs that could redefine neurological treatment and enhance cognitive health like never before. This is an exhilarating time for scientists and enthusiasts alike, as every discovery holds the promise of innovative pathways to boost mental well-being and unlock new realms of human potential. The future beckons with its promise of profound insights into our greatest asset—our brain. By staying curious and embracing these advancements, we're not just spectators; we're participants in an unfolding narrative that could change how we understand ourselves and the world around us.

Emerging Technologies and Studies

As we look ahead in the field of brain research, the landscape is bustling with exciting developments that are reshaping our understanding of the human brain and its capabilities. The convergence of cutting-edge technology and neuroscience is driving innovation at an unprecedented pace. From neural interfaces that allow humans to interact with machines using thoughts alone to advanced imaging techniques that reveal the brain's inner workings in astonishing detail, these technologies are not just theoretical—they're becoming reality.

One of the most promising areas in brain research is the development of brain-computer interfaces (BCIs). These systems provide a direct communication pathway between the brain and external devices, a concept that once existed only in science fiction. BCIs are rapidly advancing, and they're already being used to assist individuals with disabilities, enabling them to control prosthetic limbs or computer cursors with their minds. As this technology improves, the possibilities are staggering, potentially allowing for seamless integration with digital environments and offering solutions for neurorehabilitation post-stroke. Imagine the doors that'll open as we learn to harness the power of our minds in ways we've never dreamed possible.

Another intriguing area of study is neuroimaging, which continues to evolve with innovations such as functional MRI (fMRI) and positron emission tomography (PET) scans. These tools afford us the ability to observe brain activity in real time, opening avenues for studying everything from mental health disorders to the effects of learning and memory. As imaging techniques become more sophisticated, researchers can create detailed maps of neural connections, termed connectomes, which may unlock insights into how different areas of the brain coordinate to produce thoughts, emotions, and behaviors.

But it's not just about understanding the brain's current state. Cutting-edge genetic research is also diving into how our genes influence brain structure and function. The burgeoning field of neurogenetics explores the connections between genetics and brain disorders, helping to identify potential treatment pathways for conditions such as schizophrenia and autism spectrum disorders. The CRISPR-Cas9 gene-editing technology is revolutionizing the way we approach genetic research, offering the potential to correct genetic mutations at their source and possibly providing a cure for certain neurological conditions in the future.

Furthermore, artificial intelligence (AI) is playing an increasingly vital role in brain research. Machine learning algorithms sift through vast amounts of data from brain scans and genetic tests, identifying patterns and predicting outcomes with remarkable accuracy. AI is also being used in conjunction with neuroimaging to diagnose diseases at earlier stages than ever before, potentially improving prognoses and treatment plans. As AI progresses, its integration into neuroscientific research could lead to breakthroughs we can't yet imagine.

A fascinating and relatively new research area is the study of psychedelic substances and their effects on the brain. These substances are now being reconsidered for their potential therapeutic benefits in treating mental health conditions like PTSD, depression, and anxiety. Controlled studies suggest that psychedelics can promote neuroplasticity, presenting a potential paradigm shift in mental health treatment approaches. This area of research is still in its infancy, but the preliminary results are encouraging and could redefine how we approach psychiatric care.

Neurofeedback technology is also gaining traction in research for its applications in promoting mental health and cognitive agility. By providing real-time feedback on brain activity, individuals can learn to self-regulate their neural processes. This technology holds promise for treating conditions such as ADHD, anxiety, and insomnia. Advocates believe that as we refine neurofeedback systems, it could become a mainstream method for improving focus, reducing stress, and enhancing overall cognitive function.

The ethical considerations surrounding emerging brain technologies are profound, raising important questions regarding privacy, consent, and the potential for misuse. As we march forward with these innovations, it is crucial to ensure that ethical frameworks keep pace with technical advancements. This ensures that such technologies are utilized in ways that enhance human wellbeing while safeguarding personal freedoms and integrity.

As we continue to navigate this ever-evolving field, collaboration across disciplines will be key. Neuroscientists, engineers, ethicists, clinicians, and policymakers must work in harmony to integrate these technologies responsibly into society. The potential for these emerging technologies and studies to revolutionize brain health is undeniable, but they also demand a conscientious approach to how they are developed and deployed.

The journey ahead in brain research is rife with possibility. As we embrace these new technologies, we stand on the brink of transforming not just how we treat brain disorders, but perhaps even how we perceive our very consciousness and connection to the world. With curiosity and caution in balance, the future of brain research promises to be a thrilling frontier full of surprises and breakthroughs just waiting to be discovered.

Potential Breakthroughs

Every time you turn around, it seems like there's a new marvel in the field of brain research waiting to be discovered. These breakthroughs have the potential not only to change our understanding of the brain but also to enhance the way we live and interact with the world. The journey ahead promises a plethora of innovations that are as exciting as they are groundbreaking, setting the stage for future explorations into the mind's vast terrain.

Imagine a world where neurodegenerative diseases like Alzheimer 's and Parkinson's become conditions of the past. This dream edges closer to reality with advancements in early diagnostic technologies. Scientists are delving into biomarkers and neuroimaging techniques that detect these diseases long before symptoms arise. Early intervention could become a norm, with personalized therapeutic strategies tailored to each individual's genetic makeup. It's a world where we tackle these conditions head-on, armed with the knowledge and precision that modern science affords.

Another area ripe for breakthrough is the integration of artificial intelligence (AI) and machine learning with neuroscience. These technologies promise to revolutionize how we process and interpret the vast amounts of data generated daily by brain research. AI could potentially uncover patterns and parallels in cognitive function and brain disorders that were previously invisible to the human eye. This fusion of neural understanding and AI might not only improve diagnostic precision but also pave the way for innovative treatments that could redefine cognitive health care.

The potential of brain-computer interfaces (BCIs) holds another promise on the horizon. These interfaces could bridge the gap between digital technology and human thought, effectively translating brain signals into electronic commands. Imagine people with motor disabilities gaining newfound ease of mobility through mind-controlled prosthetics, or perhaps a world where your thoughts can directly interface with computers, allowing effortless communication and control of various devices. The implications are vast—reshaping communication, accessibility, and even expanding cognitive capabilities.

Meanwhile, research into neuroplasticity and how we can harness it continues to gain momentum. As you may know, neuroplasticity is the brain's ability to reorganize itself by forming new neural connections throughout life. This capability becomes particularly significant in the context of recovery from brain injuries, learning new skills, or adapting to new environments. Scientists are exploring how specific activities, therapies, and even pharmacological agents can enhance neuroplasticity, potentially accelerating rehabilitation and promoting lifelong cognitive resilience.

In the realm of psychopharmacology, novel substances are being investigated for their potential to significantly impact mental health treatments. The reemergence of psychedelic research for therapeutic purposes is one such area. Substances like psilocybin and MDMA show promise in treating conditions such as depression, PTSD, and anxiety, when administered in controlled, clinical settings. The healing potential of these compounds could unlock new methods for treating psychological disorders that have long resisted conventional therapies.

There is also fascinating work in the field of genetic research, where scientists explore how our genes influence cognitive function and susceptibility to various brain-related conditions. The rise of CRISPR and other gene-editing technologies promises advancements in understanding and potentially correcting genetic components linked to neurological disorders. It invites a future where preventive measures and personalized medicine align seamlessly to promote optimal brain health.

Looking towards the future, the expansion of our knowledge about the gut-brain axis is set to revolutionize the field of brain health. The symbiotic relationship between our gut microbiota and brain function is a burgeoning area of study that promises to alter how we comprehend mood disorders, cognition, and general brain-health conditions. By understanding this intricate communication network, innovative treatments focusing on dietary interventions and gut flora modification could emerge as pivotal players in cognitive health regulation.

You can't talk about potential breakthroughs without mentioning the continuous advancements in non-invasive brain stimulation techniques. Technologies such as transcranial magnetic stimulation (TMS) or transcranial direct current stimulation (tDCS) are not only enhancing our understanding of brain circuitry but also providing promising therapeutic effects for various neurological and psychiatric disorders. As these technologies become more refined, their efficacy for cognitive enhancement and therapeutic use could be magnified significantly.

Furthermore, the exploration of consciousness and the underlying neuronal processes promises to unlock new philosophical and practical insights. The question of what it means to be conscious continues to challenge scientists and philosophers alike. Breakthroughs in this sphere could reshape everything from ethics to artificial intelligence, leading to profound implications for how we interact with each other and machines.

The promise of future discoveries in brain research is a beacon of hope. As we accelerate towards new understandings and capabilities, the potential to reshape human experience grows. With each unveiling, the boundaries of what we can achieve with our minds expand, pushing the limits of cognition, healing, and human augmentation. It's an exhilarating era, full of promise, where each step forward reverberates with the possibility of a healthier, more connected, and enlightened society.

Chapter 19

Tailoring Cognitive Strategies for Individuals

One size definitely doesn't fit all when it comes to cognitive strategies for unlocking the potential of our minds. Everyone's unique in how their brain functions, shaped by a cocktail of genetics, experiences, and personal goals. Crafting personalized cognitive enhancement plans is like choosing the right suit for your mind—it's got to fit well, feel comfortable, and be adaptable to circumstances. By honing in on individual strengths and recognizing areas that need a little extra love, we can create tailored strategies that are as dynamic as they are effective.

Monitoring progress and tweaking techniques is crucial, turning what might seem like setbacks into stepping stones. This individualized approach opens the door to achieving long-term cognitive health and wellness, pushing us to evolve in ways we hadn't previously thought possible. With the right tools and a customized plan, the journey to an optimized mind is well within reach, tailored just for you.

Personalized Cognitive Enhancement Plans

Creating a personalized cognitive enhancement plan is like crafting a unique roadmap for your brain's journey to peak performance. The process begins with a deep dive into understanding individual needs, strengths, and weaknesses. Everyone's brain is different, making the need for tailored strategies crucial. Imagine you're about to start a fitness program: you wouldn't follow a one-size-fits-all plan, right? The same approach applies to cognitive enhancement. It's all about selecting methods that fit your personal cognitive profile.

The first step in crafting a personalized plan involves assessing current cognitive abilities. This includes evaluating aspects such as memory, concentration, problem-solving skills, and emotional regulation. Various assessments and tools can provide insight into these areas. A detailed self-assessment or professional cognitive evaluation can highlight areas that need attention. Once you understand where you're starting from, it becomes easier to plan where you want to go.

Once you've got a clear picture of your cognitive landscape, it's time to set specific, achievable goals. These goals could range from strengthening memory recall to improving focus under distractions. The key is making them SMART: specific, measurable, achievable, relevant, and time-bound. For example, if enhancing memory is the objective, you might set a goal to remember names of ten new acquaintances within a month.

After setting your goals, choose strategies that align with them. This is where the fun begins! With a multitude of cognitive exercises and techniques available, personalization is your greatest ally. Someone aiming to improve their concentration might incorporate mindfulness or meditation, involving methods steeped in enhancing attention and presence. For another, who might be more visually-oriented, employing techniques that utilize visual memory aids might prove more effective.

Integrating physical exercise is another powerful element of any cognitive plan. Regular physical activity has been shown to boost brain health significantly. Tailoring this to your preferences is crucial. Do you enjoy running? Great, aim for consistent aerobic workouts which benefit brain health. Prefer yoga? This can enhance both physical wellbeing and mental flexibility—killing two birds with one stone. The focus should be on activities that not only benefit brain function but also bring joy and satisfaction, ensuring sustainability of the plan.

Nutrition shouldn't be underestimated in your personalized cognitive journey. It's widely established that a well-balanced diet rich in essential nutrients is critical for optimal brain function. Craft meal plans that provide superfoods known for their cognitive benefits, like berries, nuts, and leafy greens. It's about fueling your brain with the right kind of energy that keeps it sharp and ready to embrace challenges. Remember, what you eat influences how you think.

Sleep is another cornerstone of cognitive enhancement. Quality rest is imperative for the brain to consolidate memory and repair itself.

Developing a sleep routine tailored to your body's natural rhythms can revolutionize cognitive performance. Sleep hygiene practices, such as reducing screen time before bed or setting consistent sleep schedules, play a pivotal role in crafting your plan.

Emotional and mental resilience is just as crucial in a cognitive enhancement plan. Stress management techniques, emotional awareness exercises, and cultivating positivity can greatly bolster your brain's capabilities. These components help in maintaining mental balance during challenging times, ensuring that stress doesn’t hinder cognitive growth.

Social interactions play a surprising role in personalizing cognitive plans. Engaging in meaningful relationships and social activities can stimulate brain regions involved in emotional regulation and cognitive processes.

Structuring your plan to include regular social activities can turn simple gatherings into brain-boosting sessions.

Monitoring progress is vital to the success of any personalized plan. Keep track of improvements, setbacks, and changes in cognitive abilities. This ongoing assessment allows for adjustments to be made as needed. Perhaps you're not seeing the benefits you anticipated in a particular area—it's okay to tweak the plan. Flexibility ensures that the plan stays relevant and effective.

Collaboration with cognitive experts or coaches can also enhance the personalization process. Regular consultations can provide external perspectives and introduce new strategies to tackle challenges. They can help refine your plan and maintain motivation to achieve cognitive excellence.

Finally, a personalized cognitive enhancement plan is not set in stone. It's an evolving entity, one that needs continuous adaptation in response to life’s ever-changing dynamics. As you grow, your brain and its capabilities evolve, requiring new strategies and approaches. Embrace this evolution; celebrate victories, learn from trials, and remain committed to your brain's thriving pursuit.

Monitoring and Adjusting Techniques

To truly tailor cognitive strategies for individuals, it's not enough to simply set a plan and stick to it without question. The essence of adaptability lies in monitoring and adjusting techniques to meet evolving needs and conditions. This process ensures that strategies remain not only effective but also aligned with personal growth and changing life circumstances. Here's how to make that happen in a way that's both inspiring and pragmatic.

First off, monitoring your progress doesn't have to be an overwhelming task. It's about keeping track of how you're doing on your cognitive journey. Maybe it's as simple as jotting down notes in a journal or perhaps using an app that lets you visualize your progress over time. Tracking can point out what's working and what's not, allowing you to make informed decisions about adjustments. It can be quite motivating to see how far you've come, and noticing areas where you're stuck can inspire fresh approaches.

Diving deeper, there's the importance of feedback loops. These are vital to ensuring that your cognitive enhancement efforts are on the right track.

Feedback can come from various sources: a coach, a mentor, or even

self-assessments. Through consistent feedback, you can adapt strategies to better suit your needs. This kind of iterative approach not only bolsters your cognitive performance but also builds self-awareness and resilience.

But let's talk about the heart of monitoring: self-assessment. It's the process of gauging your own cognitive capacities in a climate of honesty and objectivity. Through self-assessment, you can determine if your goals are realistic and if your strategies are aligning with those goals. It's about asking questions: Am I really focusing better? Is my memory improving? By regularly evaluating how you're doing, you can pivot strategies, dropping what's ineffective and amplifying what boosts your potential.

Sometimes, the adjustments required are small tweaks, like changing the time of day you practice cognitive exercises. Other times, they might involve a shift in strategy or approach altogether. Everyone's brain is unique, and what works wonders for one person may not for another. Personalization, therefore, extends into this realm of constant adjustment. It's about finding the sweet spot where challenge meets capability, fostering growth without overwhelming the system.

With this in mind, there's a preventative angle to monitoring that's worth mentioning. By keeping a close eye on cognitive strategies, it's easier to spot signs of burnout or overexertion before they become serious issues. Stress and cognitive fatigue can be subtle and may require recalibrating how much you take on at once. Adjustments can mean easing up on certain practices or including more restorative activities like meditation or light exercise.

Moreover, technology offers some incredible tools to aid in monitoring and adjusting techniques. Wearable tech and apps can log cognitive workloads and provide data visualizations. They make it easier to see patterns you might otherwise overlook. But remember, tech is just a tool. The real work comes from interpreting the results and making actionable decisions based on what's observed.

Furthermore, seeking professional guidance can enrich this adaptive process. Cognitive therapists or coaches have insight and expertise that can help you interpret data and progress more objectively. They can offer strategies you might not have considered and provide encouragement when things get tough.

Adapting to new information is part of what drives progress; it's an opportunity to grow beyond initial expectations. This dynamic process reinforces the importance of lifelong learning and the understanding that cognitive enhancement isn't a destination but a journey. Embrace the evolution of your strategies with a spirit of curiosity and experimentation.

And let's not forget the importance of setting new goals as you reach initial ones. As you monitor progress and adjust, you can redefine objectives to keep challenging your mind. This keeps the process fresh and engaging, preventing stagnation. It's all about fostering a loop of continuous improvement—each cycle taking you closer to peak cognitive function.

Ultimately, the art of monitoring and adjusting is about personal empowerment. Knowing how to assess your cognitive state and make appropriate changes gives you control over your mental destiny. It's an individualized path, full of self-discovery and refinement. By embracing monitoring and adjusting techniques, you embark on a proactive approach to cognition, not only optimizing performance but enhancing the quality of life. The journey itself becomes a rewarding pursuit of mental clarity and resilience. With the right attitude and tools, your cognitive future is bright and boundless.

Chapter 20

Enhancing Emotional Intelligence

Boosting your emotional intelligence (EQ) isn't just about understanding others; it starts with a deep dive into your own emotional landscape.

Imagine unlocking a new level of self-awareness that allows you to navigate life's challenges more smoothly. By tuning into your thoughts and emotions, you can improve your empathy, deepen relationships, and make more informed decisions. The connection between emotions and the brain plays a crucial role in this learning process. As you work on your EQ, you're not only enhancing personal development but also giving your brain a healthy workout, much like lifting weights in a gym strengthens your muscles. Remember, EQ isn't innate—it's a skill you can cultivate and refine, offering profound benefits for both your mental health and personal growth journey. Let's gear up to tap into this rich resource and transform how we interact with the world around us, because building a robust EQ can truly enrich our lives and those of others.

Understanding Emotions and Brain Connection

In our journey towards enhancing emotional intelligence, it's crucial to explore the intricate dance between emotions and the brain. As multifaceted beings, our emotions—ranging from joy to sorrow and anger to calm—aren't just fleeting feelings but are deeply rooted in our neural architecture. The brain's role in processing and regulating these emotions is both fascinating and complex, demanding a closer look to appreciate its depth and potential for growth.

At the heart of emotion processing lies the limbic system, often regarded as the emotional brain. This interconnected group of structures, which includes the amygdala, hippocampus, and prefrontal cortex, plays a pivotal role in dictating our emotional responses and behaviors. These components of the limbic system collaborate in a delicate balance to interpret emotional stimuli from the environment, encode emotional memories, and guide decision-making. The amygdala, known for its role in threat detection and response, acts as an alert system, triggering the appropriate emotional reactions necessary for survival. In contrast, the prefrontal cortex is responsible for modulating these responses, allowing us to respond to situations with reason and empathy.

Consider how a stressful event, such as speaking in front of an audience, activates this network. The amygdala may trigger a fight-or-flight response, causing anxiety or fear. However, with practice and emotional intelligence development, the prefrontal cortex can better regulate these responses, allowing for a composed delivery instead of panicking. This capability to moderate emotions highlights the plasticity of our brain and the potential to develop emotional intelligence through conscious effort.

Emotions are not merely psychological experiences; they're also physiological. The brain communicates with the rest of the body through numerous pathways, including the autonomic nervous system, which governs our body's response to emotional stimuli. Think of the quickened heartbeat when you're excited or the queasy stomach that accompanies anxiety. These physiological responses are direct manifestations of emotional states orchestrated by the brain's neural networks. Understanding this connection equips us to manage our bodily responses, aiding in emotional regulation and resilience.

Moreover, emotions are closely linked to memory and learning, further accentuating the brain's integral role. Emotional experiences are often more deeply etched into our memories than neutral ones, thanks to the amygdala's influence on the hippocampus. This partnership ensures that these memories are vivid and readily accessible, shaping our future responses and learning. Positive emotions, such as happiness and excitement, enhance cognitive processes, improve memory retention, and foster creativity, while negative emotions, if unchecked, can cloud judgment and impede learning.

Cultivating emotional intelligence involves leveraging this understanding of the brain's mechanisms. Mindfulness practices, for instance, are proven techniques that can reshape neural pathways over time. Through mindfulness, you're training your brain to recognize emotional states without immediately reacting, fostering a more thoughtful and less reactive mind. By engaging the prefrontal cortex more actively, we can override automatic responses dictated by the amygdala, cultivating a calm and focused presence even in challenging situations.

Developing emotional intelligence also means acknowledging the social aspect of emotions. Human beings are inherently social creatures, and our brains are wired to interact with and respond to others. Mirror neurons, a discovery that has shed light on empathy, allow us to understand and mimic the emotions of those around us. This ability to resonate with others' emotions is fundamental to building strong relationships. By channeling insights from our brain's empathetic nature, we can enhance our social interactions and, consequently, our emotional intelligence.

By understanding the brain-emotion connection, we're embarking on a journey to not only recognize but also influence our emotional landscapes. The potential for growth is immense, with the brain's plasticity offering a fertile ground for cultivating emotional intelligence. As we gain more insight, we forge a path toward more balanced, empathetic, and enriching experiences.

This exploration fuels an inspiring pursuit: the integration of scientific knowledge with personal development. Imagine navigating life's highs and lows with a deeper understanding and mastery over one's emotions. The objective isn't to eliminate negative emotions, but to recognize and harness them as tools for growth. As we enhance our emotional intelligence, we enrich our lives and fortify our mental resilience, leading to a more fulfilling existence.

Emotional Intelligence Development

Emotional intelligence, often abbreviated as EQ, has gained a reputation for being just as crucial as cognitive ability, if not more so, for personal and professional success. While IQ can get you through the door, EQ has the power to determine how you interact with others, handle stress, and navigate complex social situations. Developing your emotional intelligence involves enhancing certain core abilities such as self-awareness, self-regulation, motivation, empathy, and social skills. Let's dive into ways to cultivate these essential skills to improve your life and relationships.

First, understanding and increasing self-awareness forms the cornerstone of emotional intelligence. Self-awareness involves recognizing your emotions as they arise and understanding how they affect your thoughts and behavior. You might have an epiphany during a moment of self-reflection or emotional assessment. Simple practices like journaling can be extraordinarily effective in this regard. By routinely reflecting on your daily experiences and emotional responses, you can start to see patterns in how you react to different situations, which is critical for self-awareness. It's like holding a mirror to your emotions—you begin to understand why you feel a certain way, which is vital for growth.

Self-regulation is the ability to control impulsive feelings and behaviors, manage your emotions in healthy ways, and take initiative even when faced with challenges. Practicing mindfulness can be an invaluable tool here. Developing mindfulness not only helps you stay calm but also allows you to remain present, offering clarity and focus when you're tempted to react impulsively. Techniques such as deep breathing, meditation, or even short pauses before responding are great strategies for instilling a sense of calm and balance, especially during stressful engagements.

You might wonder why motivation is discussed within emotional intelligence, but it's integral to maintaining a high EQ. Intrinsic motivation—driven by personal passion, commitment, and ambitions—encourages a positive outlook and perseverance. Setting personal goals and regularly reflecting on your achievements can significantly enhance your motivation. Consider using tools like vision boards or daily affirmations to keep your aspirations aligned with your actions. The key is to stay passionate about what matters and to consistently renew your drive, harnessing the energy to pursue both personal and professional growth.

Empathy is a bedrock of emotional intelligence, allowing you to understand and share the feelings of others. Building empathy begins with active listening. Often, we are so focused on our own responses that we forget to truly hear what others are saying. Practicing active listening involves being fully present in conversations, acknowledging other people's perspectives, and responding with understanding and respect.

You might be surprised by how much you learn from others when you genuinely listen, and this awareness can deepen your connections and improve your interpersonal relationships.

Social skills round out the core competencies of emotional intelligence. They include the ability to influence, communicate clearly, manage conflict, and build rapport. This is where you truly see EQ in action in group settings. Whether you're leading a team, coordinating a project, or simply working with others, strong social skills are invaluable. Engaging in group activities, whether through work or leisure, can improve your ability to connect with others. Negotiation exercises, role-playing different scenarios, and even volunteering are ways to enhance these skills in real-world environments.

A practical application of emotional intelligence skills can have far-reaching effects not just at an individual level, but also within organizations. Businesses and institutions increasingly recognize the importance of fostering a culture that prioritizes EQ. Teams with high emotional intelligence tend to have better collaboration, improved conflict resolution abilities, and higher levels of overall productivity. Therefore, laying the foundation for emotional intelligence isn't just beneficial personally; it's a strategy for organizational success as well.

Don't overlook the role feedback plays in the development of emotional intelligence. Constructive feedback helps you recognize areas for improvement, offering insights that you might not see on your own.

Accepting feedback and acting upon it shows a strong commitment to personal growth. When you cultivate your emotional intelligence, you might even become that positive influence in your teams, guiding others on how to manage their emotions and interactions better.

Certain life experiences naturally offer opportunities for enhancing emotional intelligence. Consider how personal challenges and setbacks can pivot your learning curve. Often, adversity tests your emotional responses. These instances can teach resilience, a pioneer in preserving emotional balance. It provides that inner stability when the world around you seems turbulent, enabling you to bounce back stronger than before.

In summary, while developing emotional intelligence may seem daunting at first, the benefits are profound and widespread. As you grow your EQ, you'll find yourself enjoying richer relationships, achieving greater personal fulfillment, and unlocking new potential both in your personal and professional endeavors. Remember, growth is a journey, not a destination. Embrace the process with curiosity and an open heart, knowing that with each step, you're building a better version of yourself.

Chapter 21

The Role of Genetics in Brain Health

When we think about brain health, genetics plays a pivotal role, guiding how our brains develop and function. While we often can't choose our genetic makeup, understanding it can empower us to make better lifestyle choices that enhance cognitive function. Genes can dictate predispositions to certain mental health conditions, yet they don't tell the whole story.

Epigenetics, the study of how behaviors and environment affect gene expression, opens up the exciting possibility that we can influence our genetic legacy. By adopting brain-healthy habits, like balanced nutrition and regular exercise, we can potentially modify the expression of genes related to brain health. This interconnectedness between our genetic blueprint and our daily actions not only unveils new dimensions of cognitive empowerment but also inspires a proactive approach to nurturing our mental landscape. Through science, we're beginning to navigate this complex genetic terrain, turning potential genetic hurdles into opportunities for cognitive resilience and growth.

Genetic Predispositions and Cognitive Function

When we talk about brain health, genetics is like a hidden foundation, quietly influencing our cognitive function. Some people are born with certain genetic traits that give them an edge in areas like memory or problem-solving. For others, genes might predispose them to learning difficulties or cognitive challenges. While genetics isn't destiny, it does set the stage for how each person's brain might perform or face hurdles.

The human genome is a complex map filled with codes and instructions, some of which directly impact cognitive function. Genes like *COMT* and *BDNF* have been a focal point for researchers. These genes play roles in neurotransmitter regulation and neuroplasticity, respectively, which are crucial for cognitive abilities. Interestingly, variations in these genes can lead to differences in how we process information, remember, and learn.

Despite these genetic influences, it's essential to remember that our brains are not static. They're capable of change through experiences and lifestyle choices. This adaptability is known as neuroplasticity, a topic we've delved into earlier. This means that even if your genetic predispositions aren't in your favor, environmental factors and personal efforts can still significantly shape your cognitive functions.

Consider intelligence, for instance. While it's tempting to attribute high IQ entirely to genetic makeup, studies have shown that upbringing and educational opportunities play a huge role too. The interplay between genes and environment highlights the importance of nurturing one's brain through continuous learning and mental challenges. It's a dance between nature and nurture.

Moreover, genetics can influence more than just our intelligence or memory. They can affect everything from personality traits to the risk of mental illnesses like depression or Alzheimer's disease. These influences add another layer of complexity to our understanding of brain health.

However, with advancements in gene-editing technologies and personalized medicine, we're on the brink of new ways to mitigate these genetic risks.

Now, let's reflect on some inspiring stories. Many renowned individuals, scientists, artists, and pioneers in various fields have confronted genetic predispositions along their journeys. Whether it's overcoming a learning disability or leveraging their inherent strengths, these stories illustrate the power of persistence, innovation, and the desire to push beyond genetic 'limitations'.

What's more, understanding our genetic background can be empowering. Genetic testing is more accessible than ever, providing insights into one's cognitive predispositions. Such information can help tailor learning methods, focus on strengths, or take proactive measures against potential cognitive declines. It can illuminate paths toward optimal cognitive health, guiding both everyday decisions and overarching life strategies.

However, we should also temper our approach with caution. The risk of over-attributing behaviors or outcomes solely to genetics is real. It's crucial to maintain a balanced perspective, recognizing that genetics is one piece of a larger puzzle that includes lifestyle, habits, environment, and personal determination.

Being aware of genetic predispositions doesn't just stop at understanding. It offers an opportunity to engage with them actively, using them as a springboard toward personal development. It encourages us to ask, "How can I work with what I have?" rather than resigning to perceived limitations. This mindset can drive motivated individuals to optimize their cognitive potential.

It's a journey of continual learning and adaptation. Encouraging environments, tailored cognitive exercises, and even dietary adjustments can all contribute to harnessing and enhancing our genetic potential.

Ultimately, while we can appreciate the role of genetics in cognitive function, we must stay inspired and proactive about brain health.

The future holds promise, as emerging research and technologies continue to unfold new insights into genetics and brain function. In time, we hope to understand fully not only the "why" behind our genetic predispositions but also the "how" in utilizing these insights for maximum benefit, paving the way for healthier, more fulfilling cognitive lives.

Epigenetic Influence on Brain Health

The role of genetics in brain health is a fascinating area that is constantly evolving. While we often think of our genetic code as a fixed blueprint, it's important to recognize that our genes are only part of the story. Enter the field of epigenetics, a realm that bridges the gap between genetic predispositions and environmental influences. It's a dynamic interplay that takes genetic potential and molds it with the choices we make and the environments we inhabit.

Epigenetics involves chemical modifications to DNA and histone proteins that can activate or silence genes without altering the genetic code itself.

These changes happen due to lifestyle factors such as diet, stress, and physical activity. It's as if our genes have a dimmer switch—a fascinating concept that emphasizes the power of lifestyle and environment on our brains. Imagine having the ability to turn certain genes up or down based on how you live your life. Incredible, right?

One of the prominent ways epigenetics influences brain health is through the regulation of neuroplasticity—the brain's remarkable ability to adapt and reorganize. Epigenetic changes can enhance or impede neuroplasticity, affecting learning, memory, and even emotional regulation. In essence, how we experience and respond to our environment can reshape our brain's architecture at a molecular level.

Stress, for instance, can lead to epigenetic modifications that heighten our vulnerability to mental health conditions such as anxiety and depression. Conversely, positive lifestyle choices like regular exercise and a nutritious diet have been shown to foster beneficial epigenetic changes.

Studies suggest that these changes can promote resilience against cognitive decline as we age. It's empowering to know that our daily choices have such profound effects on our genetic expressions.

Take exercise, for example. Aerobic activity doesn't just benefit the heart and muscles; it induces epigenetic changes that promote the creation of new neurons in the brain, a process known as neurogenesis. These new neurons contribute to improved cognitive function and may protect against neurodegenerative diseases. It's a compelling reminder that leading an active lifestyle is crucial for maintaining brain health.

Nutrition also plays a significant role in epigenetic regulation. Diets rich in antioxidants, omega-3 fatty acids, and polyphenols help maintain cognitive function and mental clarity. They support the expression of genes that protect neurons from oxidative stress, which is a significant factor in cognitive decline. It's not just about feeding the body but nurturing the mind as well.

The intriguing part is that some of these epigenetic changes can be inherited. This means the choices we make today might not only impact our health but also the health of future generations. It reminds us of our responsibility not just to ourselves, but also to those who come after us. We are custodians of the legacy we leave behind, influencing health trends spanning generations.

Research in this area is still in its infancy, with many questions left to explore. How can we optimize our environment for the best epigenetic outcomes? What specific lifestyle interventions can most profoundly shape our brain health? As science progresses, we anticipate groundbreaking discoveries that will further underscore the power of epigenetics.

While genetic predispositions set the stage, epigenetics and our environmental interactions are the actors, directors, and playwrights of our brain's ongoing story. It's a narrative that each of us can influence through the choices we make every day. This blend of biology and lifestyle provides a hopeful message: while we may be born with certain genetic traits, we are not helpless. By making informed decisions, we can cultivate a vibrant mental landscape, rich with possibility and growth.

In conclusion, understanding the epigenetic influence on brain health opens a portal to proactive living. It challenges the notion of destiny from birth and empowers us with the knowledge that our choices shape our genetic expressions and brain vitality. As you embark on your journey to maintaining and enhancing brain health, remember the powerful duo of genetics and epigenetics. Together, they weave the intricate tapestry that defines each individual's cognitive destiny. By leveraging this knowledge, you can become the architect of your cognitive evolution, crafting a life that maximizes not only longevity but the quality of every thought and experience.

Chapter 22

Cognitive Impacts of Drug Use and Recovery

Drug use can cast long shadows over the brain's landscape, reshaping pathways and altering cognitive function, often leading to impairments in memory, attention, and decision-making. The toll is profound, but recovery is a journey of hope and transformation. As individuals navigate this path, neuroplasticity plays a pivotal role, offering a remarkable potential for cognitive rejuvenation. Engaging in rehabilitation strategies, such as cognitive-behavioral therapy and mindfulness practices, fosters new neural connections and can gradually restore cognitive abilities. This journey isn't just about regaining lost ground—it's also about building resilience, nurturing mental clarity, and rediscovering one's potential for personal growth. By embracing recovery, individuals can not only reclaim their mental faculties but also enhance them, proving that the mind can recover and thrive even after profound challenges.

Effects of Substance Abuse on Brain Function

Our brains are marvels of complexity, but they're also surprisingly fragile. Substance abuse, in its many forms, has a profound impact on brain function, altering the delicate balance of chemicals and neural pathways that facilitate everything from memory to emotion. The story isn't just one of harm; it's also about understanding the resilience and adaptability inherent in our brain's design.

Let's start with the basics. Substances—be they alcohol, illicit drugs, or even prescription medications taken incorrectly—interact with the brain's communication system. Neurotransmitters, the chemical messengers of our brain, are often the primary targets. For instance, prolonged alcohol abuse disrupts the balance of neurotransmitters, leading to issues with mood regulation, decision-making, and even basic motor skills.

Consider dopamine, a neurotransmitter that plays a critical role in how we feel pleasure. Many substances, like cocaine and methamphetamine, hijack the dopamine system, flooding it with artificially high levels of this chemical. The initial high felt by users is intense but short-lived, often leading to compulsive use in a desperate attempt to recreate those fleeting moments of euphoria. Over time, the brain's natural ability to produce dopamine diminishes, making users feel dull and unmotivated without the drug—a phenomenon known as anhedonia.

But it's not just about neurotransmitters. The structure of the brain itself can change. Chronic use of some substances can lead to shrinkage in critical areas. For example, the prefrontal cortex, responsible for decision-making and impulse control, is often compromised in

individuals with long-term substance abuse issues. Studies show decreased gray matter volume in users of substances like alcohol and cannabis, which correlates with cognitive impairments.

Memory is particularly susceptible. Substances like benzodiazepines can directly impact short-term memory, turning fogginess into a frequent state of mind. Prolonged abuse may even lead to memory disorders reminiscent of dementia. Alcohol, in excess, can result in Wernicke-Korsakoff syndrome, a severe memory disorder associated with thiamine deficiency.

Let's not forget about the effects on emotional regulation. Many substances alter the limbic system, the brain's emotional epicenter. This can lead to exaggerated emotional responses, anxiety, and depression. Over time, the ability to regulate emotions becomes compromised, often leaving individuals stuck in a loop of substance use as a misguided attempt to self-medicate.

For many, the focus is on the toll that drugs take on the brain, but it's equally important to highlight the brain's ability to bounce back. Thanks to neuroplasticity, our brains possess an incredible ability to adapt and heal. Removing the offending substance can, over time, lead to noticeable improvements in cognitive function and emotional resilience. However, the journey of recovery is often intricate and demands a well-rounded approach that combines medical, psychological, and social resources.

Recovery starts by addressing the physical devastation. Detoxification, although often unpleasant, is the first step in resetting the brain's chemical balance. It's during this phase that the brain begins the arduous task of rebuilding its natural pathways, a process supported by therapies that include cognitive behavioral therapy (CBT) or mindfulness practices.

The brain's plastic nature continues to astonish researchers. With sustained efforts in rehabilitation, it often regains lost functions, although the timeline varies significantly among individuals. Engaging in cognitive exercises, adopting a nutritious diet rich in omega-3 fatty acids, and ensuring regular physical activity can accelerate cognitive recovery and restoration.

Long-term success in overcoming substance abuse involves embracing holistic health approaches that foster ongoing brain health. Consider incorporating mindfulness and meditation into daily routines. These practices foster mental clarity and emotional balance, helping to break the cycle of stress-induced drug cravings.

And let's not underestimate the power of support networks. Establishing meaningful social connections and participating in recovery groups can act as both motivation and reinforcement in the journey to cognitive resilience post-abuse. These bonds provide much-needed emotional support and accountability, reducing the chances of relapse.

Today's cutting-edge research is unlocking new possibilities for aiding recovery. The growing field of neurogenesis, for example, highlights how focused efforts can promote the growth of new neurons in adult brains. Brain-training programs, targeted therapies, and even emerging pharmacological aids are expanding the toolkit available to those committed to reclaiming their cognitive health.

Understanding the effects of substance abuse on brain function isn't just about detailing the devastation; it's also about appreciating the brain's capacity for healing and renewal. With support, perseverance, and access to resources, the journey to recovery can open doors to a healthier, more fulfilling life.

Approaches for Recovery and Rehabilitation

Recovering from the cognitive impacts of drug use isn't just a linear process; it's a complex journey that demands a multifaceted approach. The brain, with its remarkable capacity for healing, deserves strategies that accommodate its intricacies. People often think of rehabilitation as a one-size-fits-all program, but in reality, personalized strategies are more effective. Each person's path to recovery can be a trail of individual steps, pivoting on personal experiences and specific substances involved.

One of the fundamental pillars of recovery is understanding how the brain can bounce back using its inherent neuroplasticity. Yes, the same concept that bolsters lifelong learning and creativity also plays a crucial role in rehabilitation. Neuroplasticity allows the brain to rewire itself, forming new connections that can compensate for those damaged by substance abuse. This is the scientific cornerstone upon which many rehabilitation strategies are built.

Therapeutic interventions are an indispensable part of the recovery process. Cognitive Behavioral Therapy (CBT), for instance, is a structured approach that helps individuals reshape thought patterns. It focuses on breaking the cycle of addiction by modifying distorted thinking and establishing new behavioral patterns. Therapies like these are not just about abstaining from substances but are instrumental in long- term recovery as they facilitate understanding and redefining responses to emotional triggers.

In addition to structured therapies, mindfulness and meditation prove to be valuable allies. These practices help in enhancing brain function by promoting relaxation and reducing stress. By fostering a present-moment awareness, they encourage sufferers to detach from the cravings and chaos drug use brings. Research shows that regular meditation can increase gray matter in regions related to emotion regulation and may even help reverse drug-related cognitive deficits.

Nutrition plays a much-underestimated role in cognitive recovery. Certain nutrients can aid in the restoration of neurotransmitter balance and improve brain function. Omega-3 fatty acids, antioxidants, and complex carbohydrates are more than just buzzwords; they are vital components that support cognitive repair. By integrating brain-boosting foods into daily diets, individuals can enhance their brain's ability to recover from substance abuse.

Physical exercise is another potent tool in the rehabilitation toolkit. Engaging in regular aerobic or strength-training routines can stimulate neurogenesis and improve mood by boosting the production of endorphins. Structured exercise programs tailored to individual preferences can aid in sustaining motivation and encouraging a healthy lifestyle — both critical components for cognitive healing.

For some, the journey of recovery might also benefit significantly from peer support and community involvement. Participating in group therapy or attending support meetings like those facilitated by Alcoholics Anonymous or Narcotics Anonymous introduces a vital social element. Sharing experiences, finding communal support, and fostering accountability help reinforce healthy cognitive patterns and mitigate feelings of isolation that often accompany addiction. Moreover, building these social connections can fortify mental resilience.

Yet, we can't overlook the importance of medical support. Sometimes, medical interventions are required to address withdrawal symptoms or co-occurring mental health conditions like depression or anxiety.

Medications that address these issues can be critical, especially in the early stages of recovery, ensuring that individuals can focus on the cognitive and behavioral aspects of their rehabilitation.

Moreover, ongoing assessment and adaptation of recovery strategies are paramount. Recovery isn't static; it's a dynamic process requiring flexibility. Regular check-ins with healthcare professionals ensure that the approaches are still relevant and effective. This continuous loop of feedback and adjustment maximizes the potential for successful, sustained recovery.

Prevention of relapse is another crucial aspect. Developing coping strategies that allow individuals to deal with triggers without resorting to substance use is a significant skill. Techniques such as grounding exercises, deep breathing, or even engaging in a quick, pleasurable activity can redirect focus away from negative thoughts, offering an immediate, drug-free way to deal with stress or temptation.

Lastly, technology is beginning to play a role in supporting drug recovery and rehabilitation. Apps offering guided meditation, tools for managing cravings, or forums for peer support place resources at individuals' fingertips, allowing them to integrate recovery practices into everyday life with ease. As technology advances, its potential to aid in recovery will only increase, providing timely support and guidance right when it's needed.

Rehabilitation and recovery from the cognitive impacts of drug use may seem daunting, but armed with the right approaches, the journey can become not just manageable but transformative. Everyone's path will differ, but with persistence and the right support, the brain's remarkable capacity for renewal can help illuminate a way forward.

Chapter 23

Influence of Environment on Cognitive Health

Your surroundings can do wonders for your cognitive well-being, shaping your mental performance and overall happiness in ways you might not even realize. Everything from the air you breathe and the noise levels you experience to the company you keep creates an environment that's either conducive to brain health or a barrier to it. Paying attention to lighting, temperature, and even the colors that surround you can enhance your focus and creativity. It's about more than just aesthetics; it's about crafting a space that supports your brain's ability to adapt and thrive. With a few mindful adjustments, you can make choices that might seem trivial but could significantly boost your cognitive performance. So, look around—your environment might just be a silent partner in your journey toward mental clarity and resilience.

Creating a Brain-Healthy Environment

Building an environment that supports cognitive health is like setting up a fertile garden for the mind. Everything surrounding us, from the colors on our walls to the sounds in our homes, plays a part in shaping our brain's function. Just as a cluttered space can cloud our thoughts, a stimulating environment can spark creativity and clarity. Let's delve into creating spaces that not only maintain but also elevate our brain's health.

First, it's essential to consider the sensory aspects of our environments. Bright, natural light has been shown to boost mood and energy levels. In contrast, dim or artificial lighting can cast a shadow over our motivation and focus. Therefore, maximizing natural light in your spaces or using daylight-mimicking bulbs can support better cognitive function. Imagine working in a room that's bathed in warm sunlight—it's invigorating and inspiring, right? And while we're on the subject, think about color. Cool hues, like blues and greens, have a calming effect, while warmer shades can invigorate and inspire. Choose colors that resonate with the emotions you wish to evoke.

Along with visual stimuli, auditory factors also influence our cognition. Noise pollution can wreak havoc on our ability to concentrate. At home or work, you can manage auditory distractions by using soundproofing elements or noise-canceling headphones. Alternatively, some find solace in nature sounds or certain types of music—they can be powerful tools for enhancing focus and creativity. The trick is to find what works best for you. Are you more productive with a silent environment, or does a gentle rain soundscape set the perfect tone?

The organization is yet another vital element. An orderly environment reduces cognitive load, enabling our brains to process information more efficiently. Rooms should be free from clutter; everything should have its place. Decluttering not only clears the space but clears the mind as well, allowing for improved concentration and reduced stress. How liberating is that feeling when you've just finished tidying up a messy desk, and suddenly ideas start flowing more freely?

Let's not overlook the role of air quality in our environments. The brain uses oxygen to function optimally, and poor air quality can impair cognitive performance and induce fatigue. Indoor plants are not just aesthetic: certain types, like spider plants and peace lilies, purify the air, increasing oxygen levels and reducing toxins. Imagine a room adorned with vibrant plants—doesn't it feel healthier and more refreshing?

Temperature control is another factor that often goes unnoticed. Rooms that are too hot or cold can be distracting and uncomfortable, undermining our ability to focus on tasks. Studies suggest that an optimal temperature for productivity is around 68-72°F (20-22°C). You could think of it as setting your personal thermostat not just for comfort but also for mental acuity.

Social elements also play a significant role in our cognitive environment. Creating a space where positive interactions are fostered can stimulate brain health. Whether it's a cozy living room designed for intimate conversations or a collaborative workspace that encourages teamwork, these settings promote socialization and cognitive engagement.

Communities thrive on connection, and when we cultivate environments that support this, we nourish our brains.

Moreover, technology use should be considered when developing a brain- healthy environment. Screens are pervasive, and while they offer connection and entertainment, overexposure can lead to eye strain, disrupted sleep patterns, and decreased attention spans. Setting boundaries, like device-free zones or scheduled screen breaks, can mitigate these effects. How about establishing a tech-free sanctuary in your home, a place where books replace screens and mindfulness is the main practice?

Personalization also cannot be overstated. Personal touches in your space, such as photographs, achievements, or mementos from travels, can be sources of inspiration and joy. These elements can invoke positive memories and emotions, acting as mental anchors in our ever-busy lives. Have you ever glanced at a family photo on your desk during a stressful day and found it calming?

Lastly, continuous adaptation is crucial because our needs change over time. Spaces should evolve with us, accommodating new interests, activities, and technologies. An environment that was once perfect might need tweaking to include a home exercise area or a new hobby corner.

Regular assessment of your surroundings can ensure they still meet your cognitive and emotional needs.

In conclusion, creating a brain-healthy environment is about balancing the elements around us to foster optimal cognitive function. It's not just about what's in our heads, but also what's around us. When we invest time and effort into curating spaces that nurture our minds, we are, in essence, planting seeds for a richer, more fulfilling cognitive life. So, consider your surroundings—how can they be tuned to better serve your mind's potential?

Minimizing Environmental Risks

Environmental factors play a significant role in shaping our cognitive health. It's often said that our surroundings can either serve as a sanctuary or a stressor for our minds. While it's true that we can't control every aspect of our environment, there are practical steps we can take to minimize potential risks and enhance our cognitive well-being.

Let's start with air quality. Recent studies show that polluted air is more than just a respiratory concern—it's linked to cognitive decline as well. Breathing in clean air may seem like an obvious need, but it's often one that's easily disregarded. You might consider investing in air purifiers, especially if you live in an urban area where pollution levels are high. Even simple acts like adding air-purifying plants to your home can make a big difference.

Sound pollution is another overlooked environmental threat to cognitive health. Constant exposure to loud or disruptive noises—like traffic, construction, or even a noisy neighbor—can impair concentration and even lead to cognitive fatigue. Investing in soundproofing options such as heavy curtains or noise-canceling headphones can provide a much-needed respite and allow your brain a chance to rejuvenate.

Water quality is also essential for cognitive function. Contaminated water can lead to various health issues, some of which might impact the brain. Ensuring you have access to clean drinking water is crucial. This can be achieved by using water filters to reduce exposure to harmful contaminants.

One of the invisible culprits affecting cognitive health is exposure to harmful chemicals, often found in everyday household products. Cleaning agents, paints, and even certain plastics can emit volatile organic compounds (VOCs), which have been linked to detrimental effects on brain function. Opt for natural or eco-friendly products where possible.

These alternatives often avoid harmful chemicals that contribute to cognitive impairment. The influence of natural light on our mood and productivity is undeniable. Insufficient exposure can upset your circadian rhythms, affecting sleep quality and, consequently, cognitive performance.

Whenever possible, design your living and working spaces to maximize natural light. If that's not feasible, light therapy lamps can be a viable alternative.

Temperature control is another factor impacting cognitive health. Extremes in temperature can create discomfort, clouding mental clarity and focus. Ensure that your living and working environments are kept at a comfortable temperature to facilitate optimal cognitive function.

Green spaces offer more than just aesthetic pleasure; they offer cognitive benefits, too. Spending time in nature, surrounded by lush greenery, has been shown to reduce stress and improve focus and memory. If you can't access expansive natural spaces regularly, even a simple addition of houseplants to your immediate environment can promote a peaceful state of mind.

Electromagnetic fields (EMFs) from electronic devices are a modern concern. While research is ongoing, some studies indicate a potential risk to cognitive health with excessive exposure. Being mindful of how much time we spend on devices and incorporating EMF-reducing strategies, like keeping your sleeping area technology-free, can be prudent.

Chemical exposure outside your home, such as pesticides, can be minimized by consuming organic produce. Although transitioning entirely to organic foods might not be feasible for everyone, even small changes can reduce your exposure to harmful chemicals.

Social environment traps like toxic relationships and work environments can't be overlooked. Surround yourself with positive influences that encourage growth and support mental and emotional well-being. Avoid environments or situations that serve as a hotbed for negativity, focusing on creating a supportive community around you.

Lastly, cultural factors can also shape our cognitive framework. Engaging in culturally enriching activities, such as learning a new language or exploring various art forms, can significantly bolster cognitive resilience and provide layers of enrichment that fortify mental strength.

In summary, while it's impossible to control every aspect of our environment, deliberate choices and small adjustments can collectively create a supportive setting for our cognitive health. As we tune into these environmental aspects, we empower ourselves to nurture our brain's fullest potential, leading to more rewarding cognitive experiences.

Chapter 24

Brain Health and Lifestyle Design

Crafting a lifestyle that strengthens brain health isn't just a goal—it's a dynamic journey that integrates the best choices across various domains of life. To power up your cognitive function, consider weaving together balanced nutrition, regular exercise, quality sleep, and stress management techniques into your daily routine. Imagine your brain as a thriving garden; it requires the right mixture of sun, water, and nutrient-rich soil to flourish. This strategic lifestyle blueprint doesn't call for drastic changes overnight, but rather a steady implementation of habits that align with long-term neuro-wellness. As you cultivate these elements, remember the essence of adaptability, allowing your methods to evolve as new research and insights emerge. Transforming your lifestyle for brain health is an enriching experience that paves the way for enhanced creativity, sharper focus, and enduring emotional resilience. Embrace this opportunity to design a life that's in harmony with your mind's limitless potential.

Designing a Lifestyle for Optimal Cognitive Function

In our fast-paced world, it's all too easy to neglect the crucial elements that contribute to a sharp and resilient mind. Designing a lifestyle that prioritizes optimal cognitive function isn't just about making smart choices today; it's an investment in your mental abilities for the future. Understanding how different aspects of your lifestyle, from diet to daily habits, impact brain health is the first step in crafting a life geared towards enhancing cognitive performance.

To start with, nutrition plays a pivotal role. Consuming a balanced diet rich in essential nutrients like omega-3 fatty acids, antioxidants, and B vitamins can boost your brain power. Foods like leafy greens, berries, and fatty fish should take front and center in your diet. These foods help reduce inflammation and promote neuroplasticity, the brain's ability to adapt by forming new connections. But it's not just about what you eat— when and how much you eat can significantly affect your cognitive abilities. Timing your meals to remain consistent and avoiding large, heavy meals that might lead to fatigue are simple changes with measurable impact.

Exercise isn't just for the body; it's a critical part of brain health. Regular physical activity increases blood flow to the brain, delivering more oxygen and nutrients that help improve memory and concentration. It also stimulates the release of chemicals that enhance mood and reduce stress. Integrating a mix of aerobic exercises like running or cycling with strength training can offer significant benefits. The key here isn't about spending hours at the gym but finding an enjoyable routine you can sustain over the long term.

Sleep often doesn't get the respect it deserves in discussions about cognitive function. Quality sleep is a non-negotiable pillar for mental clarity and cognitive efficiency. During sleep, the brain processes the experiences of the day, forming and consolidating memories. Aiming for consistent sleep patterns and creating a restful environment can transform how effectively you think and feel. Dimming lights, cutting back on screen time before bed, and ensuring your sleeping environment is quiet and cool can make a significant difference.

Mental health is equally crucial. Chronic stress elevates cortisol levels, leading to inflammation and decreased cognitive capabilities. Finding effective strategies for stress management, such as mindfulness, meditation, or even simple breathing exercises, can fortify your brain's resilience. Regularly taking time off from the hustle and bustle to engage in leisure activities that bring joy is another way to keep the mind functioning optimally.

Social interactions enrich our cognitive health as well. Engaging in meaningful conversations and collaborations stimulates the mind in unique ways. This aspect of life shouldn't be underestimated as social engagement can lead to improved memory and even protect against cognitive decline. Building and maintaining relationships that challenge and encourage growth is a critical yet often overlooked component of cognitive wellness.

The environment you create around yourself matters, too. A cluttered or chaotic space can overwhelm the brain and lead to distraction, while an organized, serene space promotes focus and creativity. Consider minimizing digital clutter and optimizing your workspace to enhance productivity and reduce cognitive load.

Technology, when used mindfully, can be a powerful tool for cognitive enhancement. The plethora of applications designed to train and improve mental speed, flexibility, and memory offer great promise. However, balance is key; too much screen time can lead to fatigue and even cognitive overload, underscoring the importance of regular digital detoxes.

Furthermore, never underestimate the power of lifelong learning. Challenging the brain with new tasks, environments, and information keeps neural pathways active and growing. Whether picking up a new language, learning to play an instrument, or engaging in complex puzzles and games, keeping the mind engaged in learning is integral to maintaining cognitive vitality.

Lastly, fostering a positive mindset can do wonders for your mental acuity. Optimism and positive thinking are linked to increased lifespan and reduced risk of cognitive decline. Practicing gratitude, setting realistic goals, and maintaining humor in the face of adversity provide a robust framework for mental strength.

Designing a lifestyle for optimal cognitive function is the art of balancing various life aspects with intention and awareness. It's about making small, manageable changes that cumulatively lead to significant cognitive benefits. With the understanding that each step taken toward enhancing your lifestyle impacts your cognitive health both now and in years to come, you're well-equipped to make choices that support a brain-healthy future.

Long-Term Lifestyle Strategies

When it comes to taking care of our brains, thinking long-term is where the real magic happens. While quick fixes might offer immediate gratification, nurturing brain health is akin to cultivating a garden—it requires patience, consistency, and attention. The decisions we make today about our lifestyles can have profound effects on cognitive health in the future. Let's explore how small, deliberate choices can evolve into sustainable habits that fuel both body and mind for the long haul.

One vital long-term lifestyle strategy is embracing lifelong learning. It's essential to keep challenging the brain with new information and skills. Whether it's picking up a new instrument, learning a language, or diving into hobbies you've always wanted to explore, the act of learning builds cognitive reserve. This helps the brain adapt and function more efficiently, even as it ages.

Another key element to consider is maintaining an active social life. Regular interactions with others not only provide emotional support but also stimulate cognitive processes involved in communication and empathy. Engaging in community activities or simply keeping up with friends and family can sharpen one's social intelligence and enhance overall brain health.

Diet plays a crucial role in sustaining brain health over the years. While it's important to enjoy a varied diet, certain foods are particularly beneficial for cognitive function. Incorporating fatty fish rich in omega-3s, antioxidant-packed berries, and a colorful array of vegetables can provide the nutrients the brain needs to thrive. Hydration should not be overlooked either; ensuring an adequate intake of water is essential for maintaining concentration and mental clarity.

Consistent physical exercise cannot be overstated as a pillar of long-term brain health. It promotes oxygen and nutrient flow to the brain, encourages the growth of new brain cells, and supports memory and learning. While high-intensity workouts can be exhilarating, even regular, moderate activities like walking or yoga offer significant benefits. The key is finding a type of exercise you enjoy, as this increases the likelihood of sticking with it over time.

Sleep, often considered a luxury, is in fact a necessity for brain health. Prioritizing quality sleep helps consolidate memories, manage emotions, and detoxify the brain. Creating a consistent sleep schedule and a restful bedtime routine can nudge your mind towards better mental performance. Avoiding blue light from screens before bed and crafting a calming environment can also enhance your sleep quality.

Stress management is another cornerstone of long-term cognitive function. Chronic stress can impair memory and learning, so it's important to develop strategies for managing stress effectively.

Techniques such as mindfulness, meditation, and deep-breathing exercises can help reduce the physiological impacts of stress and improve mental resilience.

In designing a brain-healthy lifestyle for the long haul, it's important to consider the environment in which you live. Your surroundings have a remarkable impact on your mental state, so take the time to declutter your space and make choices that encourage a peaceful and productive atmosphere. Simply adding greenery or improving natural light can enhance well-being and cognitive ability.

Mindset also plays an influential role. Nurturing a positive attitude and practicing gratitude can be transformative. Acknowledging and appreciating the good in life lowers stress, fostering a more resilient mental state. It's about creating an optimistic outlook even during difficult times, which reinforces the brain's capacity to adapt and grow.

Adopting these strategies in a lasting way means deliberately choosing actions that lead towards the lifestyle you envision. It involves regularly revisiting and refining your approach to ensure it aligns with evolving goals and aspirations. Remember, the journey toward optimal brain health is personal and ongoing, but the rewards of increased vitality, clarity, and longevity make it undeniably worthwhile.

Ultimately, the pursuit of long-term brain health is an investment in your future self. By weaving these strategies into the fabric of your daily life, you create a robust foundation for cognitive strength and agility well into your later years. While each person's path will look different, the intention to prioritize and nurture mental well-being is a powerful ally in unleashing your full potential. Your brain is a remarkable organ—deserve the care and consideration that will help it thrive for years to come.

Chapter 25

Evaluating Brain Training Programs

As we venture into the world of brain training programs, it's essential to know how to sift through the noise and find what truly works. With countless programs claiming to enhance cognitive function or improve memory, discernment is key. Start by identifying scientifically-backed criteria for evaluating these programs, such as the presence of peer- reviewed research supporting their claims. It's also worthwhile to look at real-life success stories and case studies that provide tangible evidence of effectiveness. A valuable program will not only promise lofty goals but will also offer practical and measurable outcomes. By focusing on these criteria, you're more likely to invest your time and energy into a program that makes a genuine impact on your cognitive journey.

Criteria for Effective Brain Training

Brain training programs have been soaring in popularity, promising everything from improved memory to enhanced concentration. But how do you determine if a brain training program is genuinely effective? It's not just about flashy graphics and catchy slogans. There's a real science behind what makes these programs tick and what doesn't. Let's dive into the essential criteria for effective brain training and explore how these elements contribute to genuine cognitive enhancement.

First and foremost, a successful brain training program needs to be grounded in scientifically-proven techniques. Without a foundation in solid research, the methods employed can easily be mere guesswork. Scientific validity adds credibility, ensuring the techniques are more than just trends. Programs leveraging established principles, such as spaced repetition for memory enhancement, have a demonstrated track record of efficacy. Studies should back the claims of cognitive improvements, offering transparency and trust to users.

Variation and diversity are key aspects of efficient brain training. Just as our muscles need varied exercises to grow, our brains thrive on challenges that span different cognitive domains. A program must incorporate a wide range of activities that target various mental faculties like memory, attention, problem-solving, and creativity. This diversity not only prevents cognitive stagnation but also enhances cognitive flexibility, an essential skill in adapting to new situations.

Engagement and motivation play pivotal roles in maintaining consistency. A brain training program that's boring or overly repetitive fails to keep users motivated. To be effective, programs should incorporate elements that engage users deeply, like gamified activities or challenges that adapt to each user's progress. This personalized adaptation ensures that tasks remain neither too easy nor too hard, keeping them within a sweet spot of being challenging enough to promote growth while also achievable enough to prevent discouragement.

Feedback is another critical component. Instant and constructive feedback helps users understand their progress and identify areas needing improvement. Effective programs offer detailed insights into performance, providing users with a clear understanding of their strengths and weaknesses. More than just scoring a game or a task, useful feedback is tailored and specific, allowing users to track improvements over time, and subsequently fostering growth.

Consistency in training is essential. Effective brain training programs encourage regular practice, akin to regular physical exercise routines. This consistency helps reinforce neural pathways, facilitating more permanent cognitive benefits. Programs that embed habits of regular use are more like to sustain long-term cognitive improvements. Reminders, goal-setting features, and progress tracking can help maintain this consistency.

Transferability is a litmus test for any brain training program. The skills and improvements achieved should extend beyond the training platform to real-world scenarios. Too often, users may see improvements on tasks within the program, but these don't necessarily translate to everyday cognitive abilities. Effective training should equip users with skills that benefit their daily life, from enhancing professional productivity to nurturing personal relationships through improved communication and emotional understanding.

Accessibility and inclusivity are pillars that should not be overlooked. Programs must be designed to cater to individuals of all backgrounds and cognitive abilities. This includes adaptive features for users who may have disabilities or cognitive impairments, making brain training an inclusive endeavor. Such access suggests that cognitive training isn't limited to a select few but available for everyone who wishes to enhance their mental capacities.

Lastly, an effective brain training program should include measurable outcomes and success metrics. Users appreciate knowing what they can expect to achieve with consistent use. Providing clear, achievable goals, with tangible metrics for measuring success, empowers users to track their progress toward cognitive advancement. These benchmarks not only foster motivation but also provide research data to further validate the program's effectiveness.

In essence, a comprehensive brain training program is more than a set of mental exercises; it's a scientifically grounded, user-centric approach to cognitive development. As you embark on this journey to enhance your cognitive faculties, remember these criteria to ensure that your efforts yield not only immediate results but also long-lasting cognitive benefits.

Success Stories and Case Studies

To truly understand the impact of brain training programs, we need to dive into the real-world experiences of individuals who have embraced these methods. Personal stories and case studies illuminate the diverse paths of cognitive enhancement, demonstrating the tangible benefits these programs can offer. They offer a glimpse into the transformative power of targeted mental exercises and strategies, enriched by the stories of resilience, growth, and achievement.

One of the most remarkable success stories features a seasoned teacher, who, on the brink of burnout, turned to brain training programs to rejuvenate her mental agility. Faced with increasing challenges in keeping up with her students' needs and administrative demands, she embarked on a structured cognitive workout routine. Through a blend of memory exercises and focus-enhancing games, tailored to her unique cognitive profile, she found herself reclaiming her mental sharpness. Her renewed cognitive ability not only improved her professional performance but also instilled a sense of personal satisfaction and empowerment.

In another compelling case, a retiree in his late sixties decided to adopt a brain training regimen to combat the creeping effects of age-related cognitive decline. With a history of forgetfulness and decreased attention span, he was determined to enhance his mental faculties. Through a program emphasizing mindfulness techniques and memory retention exercises, he experienced a notable improvement in his cognitive functions. For him, this wasn't merely about forestalling decline but was an opportunity to learn and grow, proving that it's never too late to invest in one's cognitive health.

Let's also look at the story of a college student grappling with the demanding pressures of academic life. The stress of balancing a rigorous coursework load with personal commitments was taking a toll on her cognitive performance. Participating in a brain training program, she focused on practices that bolstered her focus and concentration. By incorporating techniques such as time management and targeted cognitive challenges, she managed to enhance her academic performance significantly. Her grades improved, but more crucially, she developed a toolkit of mental strategies that served her beyond the academic environment.

For individuals recovering from traumatic brain injuries, brain training programs have also played a pivotal role in rehabilitation. Consider the case of a young athlete who sustained a head injury during a football game. Faced with the daunting task of reclaiming his previous cognitive abilities, he engaged in a specialized training program. His regimen included rehabilitative exercises designed to restore neural pathways, coupled with emotional resilience strategies to support his mental well-being. The journey was arduous, yet progressively rewarding, as he began to notice improvements in memory, reaction times, and emotional stability.

These stories aren't isolated anecdotes but reflective of broader trends observed in cognitive enhancement research. A case study involving corporate employees participating in brain training workshops showed measurable improvements in their problem-solving skills and workplace creativity. By integrating these programs into their daily routines, they reported better stress management and increased productivity, painting a compelling picture of how brain training can be leveraged in professional settings.

The success of these programs often hinges on their adaptability and customization. Unlike one-size-fits-all solutions, brain training programs that cater to individual needs and goals tend to yield the most significant results. This personalized approach allows individuals to address their unique cognitive challenges, enhancing the program's effectiveness and sustainability over time.

The measurable outcomes from these programs highlight the tremendous scope for personal development. Whether combating cognitive decline or enhancing working memory, the capacity for growth and improvement is virtually limitless when the mind is actively trained. It speaks to the resilience and adaptability of our brains, aligning perfectly with the broader themes of neuroplasticity and lifelong learning.

Moreover, the success stories and case studies underscore the importance of maintaining a holistic approach to brain health. Individuals who achieved the most notable gains often combined brain training with balanced nutrition, regular physical exercise, and sufficient rest. Such multifaceted strategies reinforce the interconnectedness of various aspects of cognitive wellness, underscoring brain health as a lifestyle rather than a singular activity.

In wrapping up these insights, it's clear that brain training programs hold significant promise for improving cognitive functions across a broad spectrum of individuals and circumstances. While the scientific evidence is continually evolving, the anecdotal success stories provide ample motivation and inspiration for anyone considering embarking on this path.

Ultimately, these stories are a testament to the human potential for growth and adaptation. Brain training programs offer a means to tap into this potential, facilitating a journey towards enhanced cognitive function and personal fulfillment. They remind us that, regardless of age or starting point, the pursuit of cognitive growth is an endeavor well within reach, driven by the power of perseverance, commitment, and a curiosity to explore the mind's capabilities.

Conclusion

The journey through understanding brain health and cognitive enhancement inevitably leads us to a profound realization: the mind is an extraordinary vessel, capable of remarkable change and adaptation. In this complex tapestry of human existence, our mental faculties dictate not just our thoughts but our entire being. As we reach the conclusion of this exploration, it is essential to reflect on the realities we've uncovered and how they can transform our lives.

Neuroplasticity, once a hidden gem of neuroscience, has emerged as a beacon of hope, showing us that our brains are not fixed but rather adaptable entities, ready to be shaped by our actions and experiences. This inherent adaptability invites us to embrace lifelong learning. We can continuously enhance our cognitive abilities, and it's the effort we put into learning that keeps our minds agile and receptive to new information.

Equally, the universe of cognitive enhancement strategies provides a treasure trove of tools that can be tailor-fitted to each individual. Whether through focused cognitive exercises, engaging in mindfulness practices, or even adopting specific nutritional regimens, we have the means to bolster our mental prowess. These strategies offer us the blueprint for constructing a vibrant and resilient cognitive landscape.

Physical wellness goes hand in hand with mental fitness. Regular exercise, a cornerstone of brain health, offers cognitive benefits beyond what pills could ever deliver. Aerobic exercises stimulate brain growth and health, while strength training fortifies the connections that keep our memories and thoughts intact. As the heartbeat strengthens the body, so does it invigorate the mind.

Moreover, we dive into the profound impact of sleep on our cognitive performance, acting as the reset button that allows our brains to process and consolidate new information. The restoration that sleep provides is unmatched, underscoring the importance of prioritizing quality rest in our daily lives. In a world that never seems to stop, giving ourselves permission to pause is an invaluable gift.

Recognizing the role of stress management and emotional resilience in mental well-being, we must arm ourselves with techniques that help buffer our minds against the strains of modern life. Building mental resilience provides a foundation of strength, upon which we can take on challenges without compromising our brain's health. Emotional intelligence, too, plays a pivotal role, bridging the gap between our mind and heart.

In the realm of focus and concentration, we see the true power of attention. The ability to quiet distractions and hone in on the task at hand is perhaps one of the most crucial skills in our fast-paced, digitally-cluttered world. As we refine these skills, we take control of our mental environment, allowing us to create and innovate with greater ease.

Memory enhancement extends beyond simple recollection. It's about building a repository of experiences, knowledge, and skills that we can draw from. The methods discussed in this book provide a toolkit for enhancing this capacity, empowering us to retain and utilize our past in purposeful ways.

The concept of the mind-brain connection invites us to delve deeper, realizing that our subjective experiences and objective brain functions are inexorably linked. It encourages us to approach life with a holistic mindset, where physical, emotional, and intellectual facets are treated as interconnected rather than separate.

Creativity and innovation, fueled by our understanding of brain function, are not just the purview of artists and inventors. Tapping into our creative potential helps us think differently—thinking differently sparks change. It challenges conventions, proposing new paradigms and solutions to age- old problems.

While aging is inevitable, cognitive decline is not a certainty. With the right strategies, we can keep our brains sharp well into our later years. A proactive approach to brain health, incorporating healthy habits and active engagement, can defy the myths surrounding the aging brain.

Social interactions nourish our brains, enriching our lives with diverse perspectives and emotional support. Meaningful relationships help navigate the complexities of the human experience, grounding us in understanding and empathy. They provide us with not just solace but also stimulation necessary for cognitive health.

In our digital age, technology poses both challenges and opportunities for brain health. We are tasked with finding balance to harness its benefits while mitigating its potential downsides. Digital detoxing and mindful tech use allow us to enjoy what technology has to offer without being its captive audience.

Optimism and positivity are not mere feel-good concepts; they are crucial components of cognitive health. Cultivating a positive mindset is akin to tending to a garden, where thoughts and perspectives bloom and contribute to overall mental robustness. Positivity nurtures mental strength and resilience against adversities.

We also recognize the complex interplay between genetics, environment, and lifestyle in shaping our brain health. While we can't change our genetic makeup, understanding its role empowers us to make informed choices that enhance our cognitive well-being. Tailoring brain health strategies to our unique profiles ensures that we approach personal development with purpose and precision.

Facing the future, we stand at the cusp of even greater discoveries in brain research and cognitive science. Emerging technologies and studies hold promise for breakthroughs that could redefine our understanding and interaction with the brain. This journey doesn't end here; it just opens up new horizons to explore.

In sum, we've traveled through a varied landscape of brain health topics, uncovering insights that are as practical as they are intriguing. The key takeaway is that enhancing cognitive function is an achievable goal, and the strategies discussed are pathways toward a more vibrant life.

Embrace this newfound knowledge, apply it wisely, and witness the transformation as you harness your brain's incredible potential. The voyage of cognitive enhancement is a lifelong pursuit, but with dedication and the tools within this book, the possibilities are truly limitless. As we carry forward, let us be emboldened by the power we've always possessed and the infinite paths that lie before us.

www.ingramcontent.com/pod-product-compliance
Lightning Source LLC
LaVergne TN
LVHW050912210926
848482LV00012B/412
9781068219313